NATIONAL *Sciences*
ACADEMIES *Engineering*
Medicine

NATIONAL
ACADEMIES
RESS
ashington, DC

T0221700

Exploring the Science on Measures of Body Composition, Body Fat Distribution, and Obesity

Amanda Berhaupt, *Rapporteur*

Roundtable on Obesity Solutions

Food and Nutrition Board

Health and Medicine Division

Proceedings of a Workshop Series

NATIONAL ACADEMIES PRESS 500 Fifth Street, NW Washington, DC 20001

This activity was supported by the Academy of Nutrition and Dietetics; Alliance for a Healthier Generation; American Academy of Pediatrics; American Cancer Society; American Council on Exercise; American Society for Nutrition; Blue Shield of California Foundation; Bipartisan Policy Center; Eli Lilly and Company; Found Health Inc.; General Mills, Inc.; The JPB Foundation; Kresge Foundation; Mars, Inc.; Nemours Children's Health System; Novo Nordisk; Obesity Action Coalition; Partnership for a Healthier America; Reinvestment Fund; Rudd Center for Food Policy and Health; Robert Wood Johnson Foundation; SHAPE America; Society of Behavioral Medicine; The Obesity Society; Trust for America's Health; Wake Forest Baptist Medical Center; and Walmart. Any opinions, findings, conclusions, or recommendations expressed in this publication do not necessarily reflect the views of any organization or agency that provided support for the project.

International Standard Book Number-13: 978-0-309-71517-1
International Standard Book Number-10: 0-309-71517-2
Digital Object Identifier: https://doi.org/10.17226/27461

This publication is available from the National Academies Press, 500 Fifth Street, NW, Keck 360, Washington, DC 20001; (800) 624-6242 or (202) 334-3313; http://www.nap.edu.

Suggested citation: National Academies of Sciences, Engineering, and Medicine. 2024. *Exploring the science on measures of body composition, body fat distribution, and obesity: Proceedings of a workshop series*. Washington, DC: The National Academies Press. https://doi.org/10.17226/27461.

The **National Academy of Sciences** was established in 1863 by an Act of Congress, signed by President Lincoln, as a private, nongovernmental institution to advise the nation on issues related to science and technology. Members are elected by their peers for outstanding contributions to research. Dr. Marcia McNutt is president.

The **National Academy of Engineering** was established in 1964 under the charter of the National Academy of Sciences to bring the practices of engineering to advising the nation. Members are elected by their peers for extraordinary contributions to engineering. Dr. John L. Anderson is president.

The **National Academy of Medicine** (formerly the Institute of Medicine) was established in 1970 under the charter of the National Academy of Sciences to advise the nation on medical and health issues. Members are elected by their peers for distinguished contributions to medicine and health. Dr. Victor J. Dzau is president.

The three Academies work together as the **National Academies of Sciences, Engineering, and Medicine** to provide independent, objective analysis and advice to the nation and conduct other activities to solve complex problems and inform public policy decisions. The National Academies also encourage education and research, recognize outstanding contributions to knowledge, and increase public understanding in matters of science, engineering, and medicine.

Learn more about the National Academies of Sciences, Engineering, and Medicine at **www.nationalacademies.org**.

PLANNING COMMITTEE ON EXPLORING THE SCIENCE ON MEASURES OF BODY COMPOSITION, BODY FAT DISTRIBUTION, AND OBESITY: A WORKSHOP SERIES[1]

IHUOMA ENELI (*Cochair*), professor of pediatrics, The Ohio State University; director, Nationwide Children's Hospital Center for Healthy Weight and Nutrition

NICOLAAS (NICO) P. PRONK (*Cochair*), president, HealthPartners Institute; chief science officer, HealthPartners, Inc.

S. BRYN AUSTIN, professor of social and behavioral sciences, Harvard T.H. Chan School of Public Health; professor of pediatrics, Harvard Medical School

W. SCOTT BUSCH, director of obesity medicine, Bariatric and Metabolic Institute, the Cleveland Clinic

CRAIG M. HALES, clinical reviewer, Division of Diabetes, Lipid Disorders, and Obesity, U.S. Food and Drug Administration

NATHANIEL KENDALL-TAYLOR, chief executive officer, FrameWorks Institute

MICHAEL G. KNIGHT, associate chief quality and population health officer; head of healthcare delivery transformation; and assistant professor of medicine, The George Washington University Medical Faculty Associates

---

[1] The National Academies of Sciences, Engineering, and Medicine's planning committees are solely responsible for organizing the workshop, identifying topics, and choosing speakers. The responsibility for the published Proceedings of a Workshop rests with the workshop rapporteur and the institution.

ROUNDTABLE ON OBESITY SOLUTIONS[1]

NICOLAAS (NICO) P. PRONK (*Chair*), HealthPartners Institute and HealthPartners, Inc., Bloomington, Minnesota
CHRISTINA ECONOMOS (*Vice Chair*), Tufts University, Boston, Massachusetts
IHUOMA ENELI (*Vice Chair*), Nationwide Children's Hospital, Columbus, Ohio
JAMY D. ARD, Wake Forest University, Winston-Salem, North Carolina
HEIDI MICHELS BLANCK, Centers for Disease Control and Prevention, Atlanta, Georgia
JEANNE BLANKENSHIP, Academy of Nutrition and Dietetics, Washington, DC
JAMIE BUSSEL, Robert Wood Johnson Foundation, Princeton, New Jersey
DEBBIE I. CHANG, Blue Shield of California Foundation, San Francisco, California
LAURIE FRIEDMAN DONZE, National Heart, Lung, and Blood Institute, National Institutes of Health, Bethesda, Maryland
JENNIFER FASSBENDER, Reinvestment Fund, Philadelphia, Pennsylvania
AMENDA FISHER, Walmart, Bentonville, Arkansas
ALLISON GERTEL-ROSENBERG, Nemours Children's Health System, Washington, DC
JAMIE GLONEK, Novo Nordisk, Plainsboro, New Jersey
J. NADINE GRACIA, Trust for America's Health, Washington, DC
KAYLA JACKSON, The School Superintendents Association, Alexandria, Virginia
JOHN JAKICIC, University of Kansas Medical Center, Kansas City, Kansas
GABRIELLE N. JOHNSTON, American Council on Exercise, San Diego, California
PETER T. KATZMARZYK, Pennington Biomedical Research Center, Baton Rouge, Louisiana
REKHA KUMAR, Found Health Inc., New York, New York
THEODORE KYLE, The Obesity Society, Pittsburgh, Pennsylvania
BRUCE Y. LEE, City University of New York, New York, New York
MONICA V. LUPI, Kresge Foundation, Troy, Michigan
KYLE MACDONALD, Alliance for a Healthier Generation, Portland, Oregon
MYETA M. MOON, United Way Worldwide, Alexandria, Virginia
STEPHANIE A. MORRIS, SHAPE America, Reston, Virginia

---

[1] The National Academies of Sciences, Engineering, and Medicine's forums and roundtables do not issue, review, or approve individual documents. The responsibility for the published Proceedings of a Workshop rests with the workshop rapporteur and the institution.

JOSEPH NADGLOWSKI, JR., Obesity Action Coalition, Tampa, Florida
MELISSA NAPOLITANO, The George Washington University, Washington, DC
PATRICIA NECE, Obesity Action Coalition
MEGAN NECHANICKY, General Mills, Inc., Minneapolis, Minnesota
ANAND PAREKH, Bipartisan Policy Center, Washington, DC
SARAH A. WELLER PEGNA, National League of Cities, Washington, DC
BARBARA PICOWER, The JPB Foundation, New York, New York
MARGARET READ, Partnership for a Healthier America, Prince Frederick, Maryland
VICTORIA ROGERS, American Academy of Pediatrics, Portland, Maine
CHRISTY N. ROSS, National Association for the Advancement of Colored People, Washington, DC
SYLVIA ROWE, SR Strategy, LLC, Washington, DC
MARLENE SCHWARTZ, The Rudd Center for Food Policy and Health, Hartford, Connecticut
STEPHANIE A. NAVARRO SILVERA, Montclair State University, Montclair, New Jersey
TRACY SIMS, Eli Lilly and Company, Indianapolis, Indiana
JESSICA SMITH, Mars Wrigley, Hackettstown, New Jersey
KRISTEN R. SULLIVAN, American Cancer Society, Decatur, Georgia
SUSAN Z. YANOVSKI, National Institute of Diabetes and Digestive and Kidney Diseases, National Institutes of Health, Bethesda, Maryland

Staff

HEATHER DEL VALLE COOK, Roundtable Director
CYPRESS LYNX, Associate Program Officer
AMANDA NGUYEN, Program Officer
MEREDITH PARR, Research Assistant
ANN L. YAKTINE, Director, Food and Nutrition Board

Consultant

WILLIAM (BILL) H. DIETZ, the George Washington University, Washington, DC

Food and Nutrition Board Liaison

SHIRIKI KUMANYIKA, Drexel University, Philadelphia, Pennsylvania

Reviewers

This Proceedings of a Workshop was reviewed in draft form by individuals chosen for their diverse perspectives and technical expertise. The purpose of this independent review is to provide candid and critical comments that will assist the National Academies of Sciences, Engineering, and Medicine in making each published proceedings as sound as possible and to ensure that it meets the institutional standards for quality, objectivity, evidence, and responsiveness to the charge. The review comments and draft manuscript remain confidential to protect the integrity of the process.

We thank the following individuals for their review of this proceedings:

BROOK BELAY, Centers for Disease Control and Prevention
SUSAN Z. YANOVSKI, The National Institutes of Health

Although the reviewers listed above provided many constructive comments and suggestions, they were not asked to endorse the content of the proceedings nor did they see the final draft before its release. The review of this proceedings was overseen by **BARBARA HANSEN,** University of South Florida. She was responsible for making certain that an independent examination of this proceedings was carried out in accordance with standards of the National Academies and that all review comments were carefully considered. Responsibility for the final content rests entirely with the rapporteur and the National Academies.

Acknowledgments

Staff thanks **William (Bill) H. Dietz,** the George Washington University, for providing his technical expertise in the preparation of this publication.

Contents

Box and Figures

Acronyms and Abbreviations

AACE	American Association of Clinical Endocrinology
AAP	American Academy of Pediatrics
ABCD	adiposity-based chronic disease
ACC	American College of Cardiology
AHA	American Heart Association
AMA	American Medical Association
ASCVD	atherosclerotic cardiovascular disease
BMI	body mass index
BRFSS	Behavioral Risk Factor Surveillance System
CDC	Centers for Disease Control and Prevention
CEO	chief executive officer
CMS	Centers for Medicare & Medicaid Services
COVID-19	coronavirus disease 2019
DASH	Dietary Approaches to Stop Hypertension
DEXA	dual X-ray absorptiometry
EHR	electronic health records
EOSS	Edmonton Obesity Staging System
EOSS-P	Edmonton Obesity Staging System for Pediatrics
FRAC	Food Research and Action Center

ICD-10	International Classification of Diseases-10
IOTF	International Obesity Task Force
LGBTQI+	lesbian, gay, bisexual, transgender, queer, and intersex[1]
NCQA	National Committee for Quality Assurance
NHANES	National Health and Nutrition Examination Survey
NHLBI	National Heart, Lung, and Blood Institute
NIH	National Institutes of Health
OCEANS	Outreach, Community, Engagement, Advocacy, Nondiscriminatory Support
RWJF	Robert Wood Johnson Foundation
SDOH	social determinants of health
SEM	Socioecological Model
SNAP	Supplemental Nutrition Assistance Program
STRIPED	Strategic Training Initiative for the Prevention of Eating Disorders
SWOT	strengths, weaknesses, opportunities, threats analysis
TFAH	Trust for America's Health
TOS	The Obesity Society
WHO	World Health Organization

---

[1] https://www.samhsa.gov/behavioral-health-equity/lgbtqi (accessed November 7, 2023).

1

Introduction

A planning committee of the National Academies of Sciences, Engineering, and Medicine (the National Academies) convened a workshop series[1] to explore the current science on measures of body composition and body fat distribution, with a focus on the strengths and limitations of body mass index (BMI) as a measure of adiposity and an indicator of health. Other topics examined were the anthropological and clinical perspectives of BMI, communicating to different audiences about BMI, and the policy implications of BMI on health care. The series consisted of two workshops held in 2023 (April 4 and June 26).

The April workshop explored the science of body composition and body fat distribution measures, with a focus on the strengths and limitations of BMI as a measure of adiposity and health. The presentations explored how different sectors and people from different ethnic groups, cultures, and life stages perceive and use BMI. Workshop presentations also examined BMI and alternative measures to assess obesity morbidity and mortality and how their accuracy affects obesity prevention, treatment, and policy.

The June workshop explored communication strategies and solutions to improve messaging around obesity and adiposity. Presentations

---

[1] The planning committee's role was limited to planning the workshop, and the Proceedings of a Workshop has been prepared by the workshop rapporteur as a factual summary of what occurred at the workshop. Statements, recommendations, and opinions expressed are those of individual presenters and participants, and are not necessarily endorsed or verified by the National Academies of Sciences, Engineering, and Medicine, and they should not be construed as reflecting any group consensus.

BOX 1-1
Workshop Series Statement of Task

A planning committee of the National Academies of Sciences, Engineering, and Medicine will organize a public workshop series featuring invited presentations and discussions to explore the current science on measures of body composition and body fat distribution, with a focus on the strengths and limitations of body mass index (BMI) as a measure of adiposity and an indicator of health. The workshop series will address how BMI is perceived and used globally across different sectors, ethnic groups, cultures, and across the life span. The presentations will also explore the utility of BMI as a measure to assess obesity morbidity and mortality, as well as alternative measures to BMI, and their effects on obesity prevention, treatment, and policy. The workshop series will also address strategies for improving communication about body composition, BMI, adiposity, and health across diverse groups and sectors, including strategies for mitigating misinformation or disinformation practices that lead to weight-related bias and stigma. Finally, the workshop series may also discuss current evidence gaps and potential next steps that advance the field.

---

demonstrated the connection between misinformation and bias and stigma about obesity; introduced evidence-based strategies to improve communication about body composition, BMI, adiposity, and health; and identified gaps in evidence and potential next steps to advance the field.

INTRODUCTORY REMARKS

Nicolaas (Nico) P. Pronk, president of HealthPartners Institute and chief science officer at HealthPartners, Inc., welcomed participants to the first workshop; Ihuoma Eneli, board-certified general pediatrician and professor at The Ohio State University and director of Nationwide Children's Hospital Center for Healthy Weight and Nutrition, began the second workshop. As planning committee co-chairs, they provided a brief overview of the Roundtable on Obesity Solutions at the start of each workshop, explaining that it engages leaders and voices from diverse sectors and industries (e.g., academia, government, public health and health care, business, finance, media, education, child care, nonprofit) to help solve the nation's obesity crisis. Through meetings, public workshops, reports, innovation collaboratives, and other workgroups, the roundtable provides a venue for ongoing dialogue on critical and emerging issues in obesity prevention and treatment and weight maintenance. It applies a policy, systems, and environmental change lens; focuses on sustainable, equitable strategies for addressing obesity-related disparities; and explores and advances effective solutions.

Pronk began with welcoming remarks, briefly describing the agenda and aims. He shared that the primary objective of the first workshop was to examine the state of the science on BMI as a measure of adiposity, obesity, and health. Because obesity is not universally accepted as a disease, the workshop focused on a variety of definitions and measures for adiposity and obesity, the utility of BMI in preventing and treating obesity, and the implications in the context of the clinic, public health, and health care policy.

Eneli welcomed participants to the second workshop, explaining that it built on the first to focus on communication strategies and solutions to improve messaging about obesity and adiposity across diverse groups and sectors and also linked the presence of misinformation with weight-related bias and stigma, cultural perceptions of body weight and adiposity, and evidence-based strategies for providers to shift their treatments to focus on health, and not weight.

ORGANIZATION OF THIS PROCEEDINGS

The proceedings follow the order of the workshop agendas (Appendix A) with each session recorded as an individual chapter. Chapter 2 summarizes Session 1 from the April 2023 workshop, which described the background and basis for the series by focusing on the different perspectives and definitions of obesity. Chapters 3–5 report on the remainder of that workshop, which included sessions on the tensions and perspectives around BMI (Chapter 3); applications and uses of BMI, body composition, and body fat distribution (Chapter 4); and a summary with steps for the future (Chapter 5). Chapters 6–10 are dedicated to the June 2023 workshop, which included sessions on communicating about obesity as it is defined and diagnosed (Chapter 6); innovations for communicating about body weight in the clinical setting (Chapter 7); ethics and trust in communicating about the intersection of body weight and health (Chapter 8); evidence-based approaches to improve communication about body weight (Chapter 9); and strategies and solutions to promote changes in perception and culture about body weight (Chapter 10). Appendix B contains biographical sketches of the planning committee members and speakers.

2

Obesity: Definitions and Perspectives

The first session in April included three presentations that provided background and a time line for body mass index (BMI) as a measure of adiposity and health and its effect on public health and clinical use. S. Bryn Austin, professor of social and behavioral sciences at Harvard T.H. Chan School of Public Health in Boston, Massachusetts, professor of pediatrics at Harvard Medical School, scientist in the Division of Adolescent and Young Adult Medicine at Boston Children's Hospital, founding director of the Strategic Training Initiative for the Prevention of Eating Disorders: A Public Health Incubator, and planning committee member, moderated and shared opening remarks. Austin explained that the planning committee sought presenters representing a wide range of perspectives and experiences to share familiar and novel research and viewpoints, consider, and invigorate a dynamic discussion.

CULTURAL APPROACHES TO OBESITY, BMI, AND NUTRITION

Edward (Ted) Fischer, cultural anthropologist, Cornelius Vanderbilt Professor of Anthropology, Management, and Health Policy at Vanderbilt University, and director of the Cultural Contexts of Health and Well-Being Initiative, kicked off the first session by stating that despite spending hundreds of billions of dollars on public health campaigns, clinical interventions, drug development, and other approaches, the rates of obesity in the United States continue to rise globally and nationally. While there is emerging science to better understand the underlying physiological processes to treat it and improve health, Fischer stated that it is necessary to also take into account structural racism and the cultural, colonial, and commercial factors that interact with metabolic processes to produce certain outcomes. He elaborated that the cultural lens in biology, medicine, politics, environment, culture, and economics and colonial patterns of exclusion underwrote institutions and frameworks.

Fischer shared that his research team prioritizes people living in larger bodies to understand their clinical care experiences, particularly when they learn about their BMI and diagnosis of obesity. He explained that the results of their research yielded three areas where cultural insights could mitigate implicit bias and improve health outcomes for people living in larger bodies if they were integrated into health policy and clinical care.

The first cultural insight is that "health is more than weight." Body size ideals are social constructs and different countries and cultures perceive larger bodies differently. He explained that modern body ideals originated from Western enlightenment (1685–1815) and colonialism in a racialized and gendered way. The astronomer and statistician Adolphe Quetelet developed BMI using the height and weight of European adult men (Eknoyan, 2008; Strings, 2019), leading to the European male body serving as the comparison group for all men and women.

Fischer continued by stating that people were ranked based on their body types; individuals of African, Asian, and Native American descent ranked lower than people of European descent. The results justified the colonial narrative and moralized body size with the body ideal of thin European men associated with self-discipline. Accordingly, Fischer added, women living in large bodies with dark skin were considered lazy and unwilling to forego short-term pleasure for long-term gain. Though entirely biased, the persistence of the moral prescription of body size in the United States represents a cultural fact, he said.

A cultural fact motivates behavior and is impressionable, based on tradition, experience, and popular sentiment, and not necessarily supported by science. It is as material and motivating as a scientific fact based on empirical data, measurement, and logic.

Fischer continued that scientific evidence does not support the idea, and cultural fact, that weight is an unequivocal indicator of metabolic health regardless of racial and ethnic background. He shared research by Venkat Narayan that suggests an alternative pathway to type 2 diabetes in South Asians in Chennai, India, which presents at a lower BMI than in Western populations (Venkat Narayan et al., 2021, 2022). By contrast, Fischer said, 85 percent of U.S. individuals with type 2 diabetes also have obesity, yet some U.S. residents with a normal BMI are metabolically unhealthy.

Fischer added that the energy balance model that explains weight gain as the result of more calories consumed than expended reinforces the cultural fact that people living in larger bodies are lazy and lack willpower.

He stated that although science has emerged to indicate complex and multilayered systems that differentiate human genetics, the gut microbiome, and the foods consumed, clinicians and policy makers have reinforced the moralization of body size, which has led to unsuccessful treatment and impractical health care policy.

The second cultural insight is "diet is more than individual choice." The U.S. obesogenic environment is shaped by global, agricultural, and industrial systems that foster market access and restrict consumer choice and consumption of processed and ultraprocessed foods. It therefore bolsters the cultural fact that people with obesity are overindulgent.

Fischer posed a thought experiment to illustrate the impact of cultural facts on the environment.

> Imagine the heat was turned "off" while away from home. Under normal circumstances, the house temperature is 75 degrees Fahrenheit, so upon return, the house is notably cold. To address this issue, the thermostat could be adjusted to increase the house temperature.

In his research, about 40 percent of people surveyed would turn the thermostat to 85 degrees or higher to return their house to 75 degrees. The remaining 60 percent of people would turn the thermostat to 75. The chosen strategy represents a cultural fact and demonstrates that people hold different beliefs and understandings of how a thermostat operates: Forty percent believed that it is a valve, meaning that the higher the thermostat temperature, the more heat is released. The other 60 percent understood that it responds and adjusts to the external temperature based on the temperature setting. Fischer reiterated that cultural facts influence behavior, so policies that aim to change dietary behaviors would be most effective if scientific and cultural facts were incorporated.

The last cultural insight is that "food is more than nutrition." From a scientific standpoint, food is the medium for nutrients to enter the body. From a cultural standpoint, the value of food relates to social relationships, love, and identity, including religious affiliation. Fischer acknowledged that the science of nutrition examines the metabolic impact of food consumption and identifies dietary components or substances that may impact metabolic processes to improve health. However, most people organize their diet based on social characteristics rather than the science of micronutrients or calories.

For example, Fischer offered, in Mayan communities in Guatemala where malnutrition is a predominant issue, mothers living in poverty frequently give their young children soda. For them, soda is affordable, indulgent, and a way to express love and care. Fischer compared the mothers' behavior to faith commitments to keep halal or kosher or consumer affinity for organic or locally produced foods.

Fischer stressed that public health campaigns that do not incorporate cultural context or that shame and blame and do not highlight the motivating factors or reasons for dietary habits will be ineffective. Culture and cultural context are quintessential to change behavior. Food and beverage companies understand their importance and influence and use them for marketing.

BMI CATEGORIES, DRUG COMPANIES, AND
THE DRIVE FOR REIMBURSEMENT

Katherine Flegal, a consulting professor at Stanford University and former senior scientist at the Centers for Disease Control and Prevention (CDC) National Center for Health Statistics, discussed the evolution of BMI categories and health care coverage of obesity. Many U.S. adults with BMI $\geq$30 kg/m^2, and many adults with BMI <25 kg/m^2, especially women, report having tried to lose weight in the past year (Martin et al., 2018).

According to a 2012 Institute of Medicine (IOM) report, prior to the late twentieth century, overweight and obesity were not considered a population-wide health risk (IOM, 2012). Flegal explained that weight loss was largely seen as a cosmetic issue, not as a health issue. She noted that there were some weight-loss drugs though most were relatively ineffective and some even caused health problems and were withdrawn from the market. As a result, Flegal said, health insurance companies did not cover weight-loss treatments, and they were not considered a medical deduction.

A 1995 World Health Organization (WHO) report outlined anthropometric measurements for normal weight, underweight, and overweight in pregnant women, infants, children, and adults and included three grades of overweight defined by BMI cutoffs of 25, 30, and 40 kg/m^2 (WHO, 1995), describing these cutoffs as "largely arbitrary." The report mentioned increased mortality with a BMI of 30 or greater but did not provide a reference for the statement. Notably, there was no definition of obesity with respect to body fat or BMI level.

Flegal read that a Roche company spokesman disclosed that part of the challenge in selling such weight loss drugs was to medicalize weight management for physicians. Two years after the release of the 1995 WHO report, the International Obesity Task Force (IOTF), with funding of over a million British pounds from the pharmaceutical industry (Peretti, 2013), persuaded WHO to hold a new consultation on obesity in 1997, said Flegal. Flegal continued, the IOTF drafted the report for the 1997 consultation and because the publication of the final report of the 1997 consultation was delayed until 2000, the IOTF paid for the publication of a 1998 interim version of the report and additionally paid for the distribution of the interim version to health ministers of all UN countries and to others who requested it (James, 2008). In 1995, Flegal continued, four scientists from IOTF also served on a committee at the National Heart, Lung, and Blood Institute (NHLBI) that established new guidelines for overweight and obesity. Flegal said that the 1997 WHO consultation report used the same BMI categories as the 1995 WHO report but changed the nomenclature from "overweight" to "obesity" for BMI levels of 30 kg/m² or above (see Figure 2-1).

Thereafter, Flegal said, national reports on BMI highlighted the prevalence of obesity in the United States based on the updated NHLBI cutoffs. However, clinicians were not reimbursed for treatment of obesity since it was not listed as an illness in the U.S. *Medicare Coverage Issues Manual*, which directs reimbursement for clinical services, she said. Flegal explained that an IOTF member who had joined CDC organized and chaired a CDC meeting about reimbursement of health care providers for obesity treatment, leading to the removal of language that "obesity is not an illness" in the *Medicare Coverage Issues Manual*.

Flegal noted that we have a definition of normal weight in terms of BMI, yet pointed out that at least half of the population in many countries, including European countries, are over the normal weight based on their BMI. Perhaps, she said, the definition of what is normal is not working.

Flegal said that Rubino et al. (2023) pointed out that the attribution of disease status to obesity defined exclusively by a BMI threshold is an

	1995 WHO Physical status report	1997 WHO Consultation, Obesity preventing and managing the global epidemic*	1998 NHLBI Clinical Guidelines**
BMI 18.5-<25	Normal range	Normal range	Normal
BMI 25-<30	Grade 1 Overweight	Pre-obese	Overweight
BMI 30-39.9	Grade 2 Overweight	Obese class I and II	Obese
BMI >40	Grade 3 Overweight	Obese, Class III	Severe obesity

FIGURE 2-1 New NIH terminology.
NOTES: *The classification is described as "in agreement" with the 1995 report; **The source of the classification is given as the 1998 interim report. BMI = body mass index (BMI units are kg/m²).
SOURCE: Presented by Katherine Flegal, April 4, 2023. Reprinted with permission.

intrinsically flawed concept and does not measure existing illness. As also pointed out by Rubino et al., Flegal continued, a blanket definition of obesity as a disease involves a significant proportion of the population worldwide. This definition could render large numbers of people suddenly eligible for claims of disability or expensive treatments. Such claims would effectively make obesity a financially and socially intractable issue (Rubino et al., 2023). Recent peer-reviewed research provides a shift in thinking from using BMI as a predictor of future disease or mortality to a clinical definition of obesity that measures existing illness (Bosy-Westphal and Müller, 2021; Rubino et al., 2023).

CLINICAL CONTEXT: HOW CAN WE MEASURE A DISEASE TO TRACK ITS IMPROVEMENT?

Donna Ryan, professor emerita at Pennington Biomedical and consulting advisor to companies for obesity management, was the third presenter. As a clinician, Ryan focuses on identifying a measure that can define obesity as a disease and tracking its progress with clinical treatment. She provides continuing medical education to clinicians on obesity diagnosis and treatment and consults with companies on lifestyle interventions, medications, and medical devices to treat obesity.

Ryan agreed with Flegal that obesity is a disease with an etiology and pathogenesis. Before 2004, she continued, it was not listed as a disease by the Centers for Medicare & Medicaid Services (CMS) and Health Care Financing Administration for reimbursement claim submissions for professional services to treat it. Ryan asserted that the tipping point for it to be considered a disease was the 2013 American Medical Association (AMA) resolution, even though several professional society white papers, position statements, and the 1998 NHLBI obesity guidelines already deemed it so (Kyle et al., 2016).

Ryan acknowledged the debate on obesity as a disease in the medical community and provided an overview of the etiology and pathogenesis for this conceptualization. Ryan introduced the Soggy Bathroom Carpet Model of Over-Nutrition-Related Metabolic Disease (O'Rahilly, 2021), which posits that given a continuous positive energy balance that compromises the body's ability to store healthy fat in the adipose tissue depots (e.g., hips; thighs), ectopic and abnormal fat stores (in and around organs) increase, leading to metabolic disease (Blüher, 2020). In the bathtub metaphor, when a person consumes more energy than is expended in physical activity, their consumption acts as the faucet, their energy expenditure acts as the drain and the extra energy is stored as fat in the bathtub. When the adipose tissue stores exceed the capacity of the bathtub, the extra energy and fat overflow to become a soggy bathroom carpet, representing dysmetabolic disease (e.g., type 2 diabetes).

Ryan explained that where the body stores fat (healthy fat storage in the hips and thighs or ectopic, unhealthy fat storage in and around organs) is determined by factors such as age, medications that instigate lipodystrophy, and hormone fluctuations in menopause. Unhealthy ectopic and visceral fat stores behave differently from healthy subcutaneous fat. Microscopically, the ectopic and visceral fat tissue exhibits enlarged cells and dying helmet cells infiltrated by macrophages that produce adipokines, leading to thrombosis and inflammation.

According to Ryan, the true definition of obesity is "excess abnormal body fat that leads to poor health outcomes." The fat's location determines the pathogenesis for complications (see Figure 2-2).

Ryan described the anatomy of epicardial adipose tissue, which is located under the pericardium and epicardium, adjacent to the myocardium and traversed by the coronary arteries. It can promote damage to the

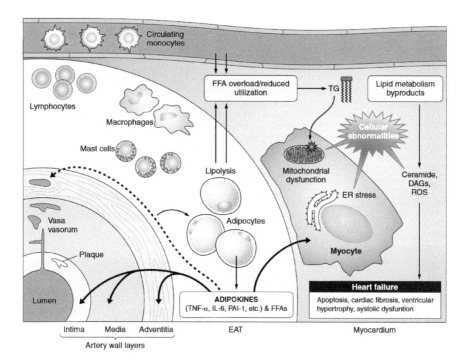

FIGURE 2-2 Role of epicardial adipose tissue in cardiovascular risk.
NOTE: DAG =-diacylglycerols; ROS = reactive oxygen species; EAT = epicardial adipose tissue; ER = endoplasmic reticulum; FFA = free fatty acids.
SOURCES: Presented by Donna Ryan, April 4, 2023. Cherian et al. (2012). Reprinted with permission.

myocardium and atherogenesis in the coronary arteries by direct exposure to adverse cytokines.

Ryan added that the mechanical burden of excess abnormal fat can also lead to disease. For example, she said, greater visceral adiposity causes intra-abdominal pressure that increases the risk for gastroesophageal reflux disease. Another example is that excess adipose tissue near the neck can constrict the airway system, leading to a mechanical burden and sleep apnea (see Figure 2-3).

Fortunately, Ryan continued, the body preferentially removes ectopic and visceral fat tissue during weight loss, which immediately benefits health. The physiology of weight loss, she reiterated, is that different tissues respond differently to different degrees of weight loss. By removing abnormal body fat, a person can reduce their risk for metabolic disease. She specified that a proportional weight loss of 5, 10, and 15 percent yields health benefits but not necessarily a BMI in a "normal or healthy range" (≤ 25 kg/m^2). To illustrate this point, Ryan noted that most participants of the Diabetes Prevention Program who demonstrated an impaired glucose tolerance and lost 5–10 percent of their body weight prevented their progression to type 2 diabetes (Hamman et al., 2006), despite still being classified as having overweight or obesity by BMI.

Ryan acknowledged valid criticisms of BMI cutoffs as a screening tool. In the clinic, some patients with a BMI ≥ 30 kg/m^2 are metabolically healthy, and others with a healthy or normal BMI (<25 kg/m^2) have excess abnormal body fat and metabolic complications. Clinical judgment, she affirmed, is essential to diagnose obesity based on evidence from measuring excess abnormal body fat by waist circumference and assessing its cardiometabolic risk factors and symptoms.

Ryan pointed out that most clinicians recognize that BMI does not assess health, although it is important because it is automated in electronic health records (EHRs), is included as a diagnostic code for overweight and obesity (E66) in the International Classification of Diseases, Tenth Revision (ICD-10), and directs insurance coverage. However, she said, only 50 percent of patients who meet the BMI criteria are diagnosed with obesity on the medical record, and only 21 percent of Medicare claims include a diagnosis of obesity, because clinicians are not reimbursed for a comprehensive spectrum of treatments associated with the diagnosis.

Ryan noted that alternatives to BMI do have limitations. The clinical setting has no reliable measure for percent of lean and fat mass. The gold standard to measure fat mass, lean mass, and location is dual X-ray absorptiometry (DEXA), although it is unfeasible for regular widespread use because of the radiation exposure. Ryan mentioned other tools, such as bioimpedance analysis, which is easy to use but inaccurate, and air displacement plethysmography (i.e., Bod Pod), which measures body fat volume but

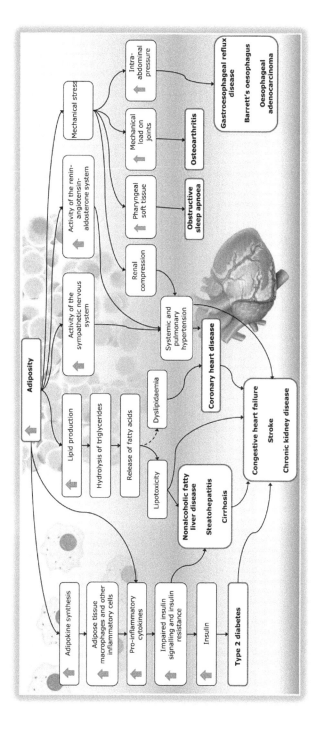

FIGURE 2-3 Growing understanding of how excess abnormal fat drives disease.
SOURCES: Presented by Donna Ryan, April 4, 2023. Wilding and Jacob (2021). Reprinted with permission.

is cumbersome, expensive, and unable to specify fat distribution. She also mentioned digital anthropometry through phone applications (e.g., Me360[1]), which is intuitive for untrained individuals to accurately determine their body fat percentage by measuring bicep, thigh, stomach, and calf circumferences, but it requires validation in clinical research. Ryan ended by underscoring the need for an additional tool to complement BMI to clinically diagnose obesity and allow clinicians to track their patient's treatment and progress.

PANEL AND AUDIENCE DISCUSSION

Following the panel presentations, Austin moderated a discussion. Fischer, Flegal, and Ryan addressed questions from workshop participants about educating students on the nuances of the energy balance model; alternatives to BMI to surveil population health; debates about the utility of BMI in the clinical setting; the origin of the "obesity epidemic"; and the intersections of racial and gender stigmas with weight stigma.

Educating Medical and Allied Health Students on the Nuances of the Energy Balance Model

Austin referred to Fischer's presentation and thesis on the racist and colonialist narrative of weight stigma and its support for the energy balance myth. Yet, she contended, the energy balance model persists in medical schools and schools for allied health care professionals. Austin asked Fischer to comment on how universities can educate students on the flaws of that model.

Fischer emphasized the importance of uncovering students' and instructors' implicit biases that reinforce scientific or pseudoscientific models. He proposed interrogating the conceptual framework for obesity to reduce bias and incorporate anthropology into curriculum, including lived experiences and examples from other countries and cultures. For example, he added, the Japanese government redefined obesity as a metabolic syndrome through additional measures for a composite to examine disease pathology, beyond body weight.

Alternative Measures to Surveil Obesity and Public Health

Austin reminded the audience of Flegal's presentation on the history and role of commercial actors in the WHO IOTF consultation report, the obesity epidemic, and the concept of obesity as a disease. Given this history, Austin asked Flegal how we can reconcile BMI's use as a public health surveillance tool.

---

[1] https://www.methreesixty.com/body-fat-calculator (accessed September 22, 2023).

Flegal responded that public health reports must clearly define their relevance and importance for public health. She recounted publications on the prevalence of obesity measured by BMI that highlighted it as a significant public health problem in the United States. According to Flegal, these reports were somewhat misleading because they were saying people had a disease when there was no reason to think that these people necessarily had a disease. The articles were well received by pharmaceutical companies and public health because the high prevalence of obesity showing that obesity is an epidemic gave them something to work with. However, Flegal said, these reports could be contributing to weight stigma and harm.

Function of BMI in Clinical Practice

Austin reminded participants of Ryan's presentation on the complexity of adipose tissue, the challenges to accurately measure it, and the recognition that BMI as an embedded measure in EHRs will persist in monitoring health. She asked Ryan, "How can clinicians avoid using BMI?"

Ryan emphasized that BMI is a screening tool and obesity is a clinical diagnosis. Furthermore, she added, it is in the ICD codes for diabetes and fatty liver disease, and patients with these diagnoses benefit from weight loss. She reiterated that the objective of therapeutic weight loss should not be to achieve some BMI cutoff. That may not be needed for health benefits. Reaching certain targets for proportional weight loss (e.g., 5, 10, or 15 percent) can produce health benefits in persons who still meet BMI criteria for overweight or obesity.

Origin of Obesity as an Epidemic

An audience member asked Flegal whether catastrophizing obesity as an epidemic originated from the business or public health sector. Flegal stated that the origin of the obesity epidemic stemmed from both sectors, as well as cultural and economic factors. For example, there is a notable cultural difference in attitude about weight between men and women. Further, people are heavily invested in these issues and put them forward.

The Intersection of Racial Stigma, Gender Stigma, and Weight Stigma

The last question from the audience asked Fischer whether the literature distinguishes between racial and gender stigma regarding weight stigma and whether one is more strongly predictive of weight stigma. Fischer admitted he had not considered if one factor was more influential than the other but said that it was a critical future research question.

3

Tensions and Perspectives Around BMI

The second session was dedicated to body mass index (BMI) and the surrounding tensions in different contexts. Michael G. Knight, internist and obesity medicine specialist, medical director at the George Washington Medical Faculty Associates, and associate chief of quality and population health and assistant professor at George Washington University (GWU), moderated and introduced the panel, which had three presentations that detailed perspectives on the strengths and limitations of BMI in clinic, more broadly in public health surveillance, and from a patient's lived experience. Knight concluded by leading a panel and audience discussion.

TENSIONS AND PERSPECTIVES AROUND BMI: A CLINICIAN PERSPECTIVE

Jamy D. Ard, professor in the Department of Epidemiology and Prevention and the Department of Medicine at Wake Forest University School of Medicine and codirector of the Atrium Health Wake Forest Baptist Weight Management Center, provided a clinician's perspective on the routine use and value of BMI in clinics and the challenges of interacting with patients with regard to BMI.

Ard agreed that BMI is a screening tool, although he emphasized the lack of a reliable method to estimate fat mass in clinical practice. He asserted that the value of BMI as a measure of health risk must be interpreted alongside other health indicators in clinical practice. For example, Ard stated, weight trajectory is a more accurate indicator, regardless of BMI. Typically, he said, only wrestlers and pregnant people are actively or intentionally gaining weight, so weight trajectory is more informative than a static BMI.

As a physician, Ard shared that it is standard clinical practice to use BMI cutoffs to determine treatment for a patient who has overweight or obesity. For example, a clinician may prescribe pharmacotherapy for patients with a BMI of 27 kg/m^2 and one or more complications related to overweight, or for patients with a BMI of 30 kg/m^2 or greater. The Centers for Medicare & Medicaid Services (CMS) provides guidance on the behavioral therapies for obesity treatment that are covered and reimbursable. Ard elaborated that Medicare beneficiaries pursuing coverage for intensive behavioral counseling and behavioral therapy for obesity must have a BMI of 30 kg/m^2 or greater, for example (CMS, 2011).

Notably, Ard continued, CMS does not cover or reimburse clinicians for intensive behavioral therapy for someone without a BMI of 30 kg/m^2 or greater. He highlighted the paradox for clinicians submitting claims for reimbursement to CMS and private insurers and using BMI as a directive for health care coverage. If a provider successfully treats a patient with a BMI of 31 kg/m^2, theoretically, they may not be reimbursed once that BMI is 30 kg/m^2 or lower.

Ard described the use of BMI in treatment allocation. Payers or employers typically do not cover treatment services for all payees or employees with obesity due to cost. Instead, he said, insurers create criteria or goalposts, and employers can choose to cover surgical treatment for individuals with a BMI of 40 kg/m^2 or higher or offer workplace wellness initiatives for all employees.

Ard reiterated the value of BMI as a diagnostic tool. It is standardized, easy to calculate, and found in the electronic health record (EHR). The challenge, he admitted, is the lack of distinction between type of fat or its distribution. As people age, he said, they lose lean body mass and gain fat mass; they can maintain their weight and BMI but have demonstrably different percent body fat. Even so, BMI is an integrated diagnostic criterion and required for treatment and reimbursement.

According to Ard, providers know that BMI means "body mass index," and the cutoffs are broadly understood. BMI is associated with several clinical risk factors, including fat mass using dual X-ray absorptiometry (DEXA) (R^2 = 0.7–0.8), depending on the population. He added that it is not highly correlated with fat mass in special populations, such as football players or sarcopenic older adults.

Ard maintained that because BMI is integrated into the EHR, the International Classification of Diseases, Tenth Revision (ICD-10), insurance treatment allocation, and indication, it is critical that clinicians have conversations with patients about it. However, he cautioned, patients do not have context or an understanding of BMI and hold various opinions, yielding both the potential to cause harm and an opportunity to educate and engage them to focus on their health. Ard commented that many patients incorrectly assume they will be healthy once they achieve a "normal" BMI. He advocated for clinicians to use the opportunity to educate patients about their health risk and the prospect to reduce it immediately by initiating weight loss. Ard also acknowledged the patients who do not believe BMI applies to them because they are not White and suggested that clinicians refocus the conversation on health by affirming their concerns and asking if losing weight could be helpful.

Ard recapped that BMI is the long-term measurement and that, although BMI cutoffs define obesity as excess body fat, the real health risk is energy dysregulation. After all, if excess fat were the health concern, liposuction or body sculpting would be the optimal treatment.

BMI: A PUBLIC HEALTH PERSPECTIVE

Cynthia Ogden, an epidemiologist at the National Center for Health Statistics, Centers for Disease Control and Prevention (CDC), and manager of the National Health and Nutrition Examination Survey (NHANES) analysis group, provided a public health perspective on BMI and discussed its strengths and limitations.

Ogden began by agreeing with Ard that BMI is a simple and inexpensive tool. It is strongly correlated with body fat at the population level and useful to observe trends over time (Hales et al., 2018). Conversely, she said, it is not a direct measure of body fat and does not capture fat distribution or distinguish between fat and lean body mass. Furthermore, the association between BMI and adiposity or health outcomes varies by ethnic group.

Obesity definitions can vary. Ogden stated that children and adolescents have different reference populations around the world, with considerable variability between country-specific charts, World Health Organization (WHO) growth standards for birth to 5 years and 5–18 years, International Obesity Task Force (IOTF) cutoffs for children aged 2–18, and CDC growth charts, with gender-specific BMI cutoffs that vary by age. U.S. adult obesity and severe obesity are defined by cutoffs of 30 kg/m^2 and 40 kg/m^2, respectively. Conversely, in China, obesity is defined by a cutoff of 28 because of an increased health risk (Zeng et al., 2021).

Ogden noted that obesity prevalence varies based on the chosen BMI cutoffs and whether height and weight is self-reported or measured. For example, trained professionals measure the height and weight in NHANES and enter these directly from the stadiometer and scale into the database. From 2017 to March 2020, NHANES results showed that nearly 42 percent of people in the United States had obesity (Stierman et al., 2021). Data from the 2020 Behavioral Risk Factor Surveillance System (BRFSS), Ogden reported, which is based on self-reported height and weight, showed only 31.9 percent (CDC, 2020). Ogden indicated that the discrepancy was due to people overreporting their height and underreporting their weight.

A strength of BMI, Ogden stated, is its epidemiological use for obesity surveillance over time overall and for different groups and geographic locations. Regardless of the chosen cutoffs, trends emerge when the same cutoff is used. Illustrating the strength of BMI, Ogden shared a graph of increasing trends in age-adjusted obesity and severe obesity among women by race and ethnicity between 1999 and 2018 (Ogden et al., 2020) (see Figure 3-1). Ogden added that it is also useful to observe changes in the population distribution of BMI.

BMI is also limited, Ogden conceded, and can mischaracterize body fat. For example, in an NHANES study of girls aged 8–19, Black girls had a significantly greater prevalence of obesity (BMI ≥30 kg/m^2) when compared to White and Mexican American girls, but no significant differences were found when adiposity was measured with DEXA scans (Flegal et al., 2010). Similarly, other research using NHANES data found inconsistent distributions of body fat and BMI for U.S. boys aged 8–19 between racial and ethnic groups (Martin et al., 2022).

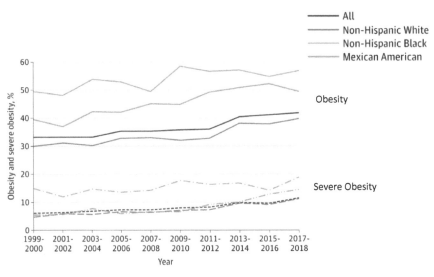

FIGURE 3-1 Trends in women show increases in obesity and severe obesity in all racial/ethnic groups.
SOURCES: Presented by Cynthia Ogden, April 4, 2023. Reproduced with permission from *Journal of the American Medical Association.* 2020. 324(12):1208-1210. Copyright ©(2020) American Medical Association. All rights reserved.

Furthermore, Ogden shared, BMI is also variable as an indicator for the prevalence of diabetes. In the U.S., obesity (BMI ≥30 kg/m^2) is more prevalent among White adults, at 41.4 percent compared with just 16.1 percent of Asian adults (Stierman et al., 2021). Even so, the percentage of Asian adults diagnosed with diabetes was similar to White adults (CDC, 2022).

Ogden summarized some key considerations for BMI in public health monitoring and surveillance. First, she said, the cutoffs vary, and among children and adolescents, different age- and sex-specific reference populations are used. Next, BMI is most useful for monitoring population trends. Third, self-reported weight is underreported and height overreported, which leads to lower BMI. Finally, Ogden reminded the audience of the variability between racial and ethnic groups concerning the relationship of BMI with body fat or diabetes diagnoses.

LIVED-EXPERIENCE PERSPECTIVE

Stacy E. Wright, a Ph.D. student in the Health Outcomes and Implementation Science Program at the University of Florida, rounded out Session 2 by recounting her experience with the Jamaican and U.S. health care systems from childhood to adulthood.

Wright opened by emphasizing the stress she felt as a child about her body and appearance and its impact on her mental and physical health. She learned early on to focus on her excess weight and not health risks. She was a competitive swimmer and ballet student as a child, but her parents worried about her body size and monitored and criticized her eating habits; despite her eating habits and appearance, blood tests verified that she was metabolically healthy.

Wright described her experience of being shamed and stigmatized and having her accomplishments minimized. She internalized comments and pseudo-compliments about her weight: "You are pretty for a fat person." Wright recalled an incident at a high-jump competition at school that shaped her self-esteem and self-worth. She was a finalist, and a spectator called her a "fatty," causing the crowd to laugh at her. After that, she refrained from activities that would put her at risk for being teased and focused on her academic work.

Wright admitted that in private, she was obsessed with fashion magazines and convinced that her life would be better in a thin body and that she would be normal. She saw reminders about the value of thinness everywhere in her environment. Stores had countless mirrors and a limited range of clothing sizes. She was teased and bullied about her size by strangers and felt intense anxiety about certain spaces and objects that could not accommodate her weight. She recalled that these experiences led her to diet for weight loss in young adulthood.

At 28 years old, she was diagnosed with hypertension, and it prompted her to improve her eating habits and increase her physical activity. She learned about nourishing foods and strived for a lower body weight range to avoid a lifetime of taking medication for hypertension. Wright lost over 100 pounds and is almost within a normal BMI range, though her weight continues to fluctuate by 10–20 pounds. Since then, she has been working with a team of doctors who are focused on her progress and health and not BMI. Her blood pressure is under control.

Wright ended by encouraging providers to seek continuing education on weight bias and discrimination, improve patient–provider communication, and approach patients as individuals with unique experiences, knowledge, and goals.

PANEL AND AUDIENCE DISCUSSION

A moderated panel discussion was led by Knight at the end of the second session. Questions from the audience to Ard, Ogden, and Wright encompassed alternatives to BMI to monitor obesity at the population level; using BMI in the clinical setting; communicating with patients about weight, BMI, and health; fostering open dialogue between patients and their providers; and using BMI as a threshold to determine treatment modalities.

Alternative Measures to Monitor Obesity at the Population Level

Referring to Ogden's presentation on the strengths and limitations of BMI as a measure of obesity, Knight asked Ogden to comment on alternative measures for monitoring at the population level. Ogden emphasized that the challenge of replacing BMI is its simplicity and affordability. Moreover, for obesity at the population level, different datasets have advantages and disadvantages. BRFSS captures state and county-level data on BMI and obesity but uses self-reported weight and height, which is less accurate. NHANES offers a national snapshot of obesity and BMI and periodically measures body fat using DEXA scans, which are accurate but require training and are expensive and time consuming.

Utility of BMI in the Clinical Setting

Knight turned the discussion to Ard's presentation on the clinical perspective of BMI and asked how clinicians could best use it. Ard reiterated that, paired with BMI, weight trajectory is essential to integrate into a clinical assessment for obesity. After a year of treatment, Ard continued, some patients return to their physician with significant weight loss, and if clinicians only consider BMI, they will likely emphasize the need to lose more weight. He argued that integrating weight trajectory tells a story. EHRs show a change in weight and BMI at each doctor's visit and could integrate with other health indicators, such as the atherosclerotic cardiovascular disease (ASCVD) risk score that calculates a 10-year risk for a cardiovascular event (e.g., stroke). Ard continued that other information could be useful to determine health-related risk, such as sleep apnea, family history, social determinants of health (SDOH), and the EHR could ideally synthesize the data for the clinician.

Communicating with Patients About BMI, Weight, and Health Risk

Knight noted the challenge of communicating with patients about BMI and health risks from Wright's presentation. He shared that in his experience, clinicians consider 5–7 factors when assessing a patient's adiposity and health risk, which can be challenging to explain to a patient versus a straightforward BMI cutoff. Knight asked Wright to comment on how clinicians can better explain their clinical judgment of BMI to patients.

Knight responded that clinicians could use layperson terms to foster an open dialogue about BMI and related health risks because patients do not have the same knowledge or language as clinicians and are intimidated. Wright suggested that they spend time with people and focus on establishing a rapport because communication is unique to the situation. She added that they could shift away from "overweight," "fat," or "obesity," which have negative connotations.

Improving the Distinct Interactions of Patients and Providers

An audience member noted the importance of individual care and the time that clinicians need to build a relationship and asked Ard to comment on what he thought it would take to train clinicians to make patient–provider interactions more positive and holistic. Ard responded that the health care system needs to change. He highlighted that insurers and payers pay providers and clinicians not to improve health but to see more patients. Providers need more time during appointments and also a more efficient way to integrate data in the EHR to understand patients over time and in the context of their health history.

BMI as a Threshold for Treatment Modalities

The last question, from an audience member, was about whether BMI should still be a threshold for treatment modalities, such as medication or surgery. Ard acknowledged that the question suggested that BMI should not be a threshold and that clinicians must use their medical judgment to understand the modality. Nevertheless, he noted practical cost issues and the cultural phenomena of thinness. Furthermore, having treatment available for everyone who could afford it would cause ethical and resource challenges along socioeconomic lines.

4

Applications and Uses of BMI, Body Composition, and Body Fat Distribution

The third session sharpened the focus on body mass index (BMI), body composition, and body fat for a more detailed examination of their application to determine obesity and health risks. W. Scott Butsch, the director of obesity medicine at the Bariatric and Metabolic Institute at the Cleveland Clinic, led the session, which had four presentations on the biology of fat and lean body mass, alternative measures to BMI and the financial implications in health care, using BMI in occupational health and safety research, and the lived experience of a person living with obesity. Butsch then moderated a panel discussion with questions from the audience.

ADIPOSE TISSUE, BMI, AND FAT DISTRIBUTION

Michael Jensen, Tomas J. Watson, Jr. Professorship in Honor of Dr. Robert L. Frye at the Mayo College of Medicine and consultant in the Division of Endocrinology and Metabolism, asked the audience to consider if BMI is a surrogate for body fat and why the amount and distribution of fat matter. To answer, Jensen gave a brief lesson in biology on the differences between lean body mass and adipose tissue.

Jensen explained that BMI and body fat are correlated, but body fat percentage varies considerably in any given range of BMI. To illustrate, he referenced his unpublished study of adults with a BMI of 20–25 kg/m², which showed that women who were metabolically healthy had double the body fat percentage (~30 percent) of men. In the same study, men with a BMI of 30–35 kg/m² also had about 30 percent body fat but were metabolically unhealthy.

Jensen provided an overview of the role of adipose tissue or body fat in processing dietary fat. Its chief function is to store enough energy for about 2–3 months. After a meal, dietary fat is broken down into triglycerides that circulate through the bloodstream and are removed and stored as body fat. Fat cells produce storage proteins to remove triglycerides from the bloodstream. Body fat or adipose tissue releases the fatty acids into the bloodstream as an energy source for other tissues. Otherwise, dietary fat and triglycerides would build up in the bloodstream, leading to poor metabolic health.

Jensen emphasized that fat metabolism is tightly regulated. When someone is not eating, fat tissue releases 1 teaspoon of fatty acids per minute into the bloodstream, circulating to other body tissues for energy. However, when adipose tissue is not functioning normally, that release is 1.4 teaspoons per minute, leading to an increased risk for hyperlipidemia and diabetes.

A predictor of poor metabolic health is the location of fat distribution in the body, Jensen continued. Visceral fat (in the abdomen) is strongly associated with adverse metabolic consequences (e.g., diabetes, hyperlipidemia), whereas subcutaneous fat (under the skin) is not. Jensen described his research that found a positive relationship between BMI and visceral fat in men and women, although women in any BMI range had less visceral fat. BMI was somewhat predictive of visceral fat, and visceral fat was somewhat predictive of poor metabolic health. However, Jensen shared that his research showed the size of fat cells is more predictive of fat cell dysfunction. Jensen's study indicated that small fat cells efficiently generated fat storage proteins for triglyceride uptake and rapidly regulated the release of fatty acids. By contrast, large fat cells were dysfunctional within any range of BMI, produced fewer fat storage proteins, and were less efficient at removing triglycerides from the blood.

Returning to BMI as a measure, Jensen stated that despite the positive relationship with fat cell size it is not reliable. Some people with a BMI within a normal range have large fat cells, whereas others with a BMI in the overweight range have small fat cells. To summarize, he said, the smaller the fat cells, the greater efficiency in fat tissue.

Jensen stated that visceral or abdominal fat is considered a predictor of fat cell size. His research found that people with less visceral fat, measured by (smaller) waist circumference, had smaller fat cells. The greater the waist circumference, the more visceral fat, and the greater the likelihood of large fat cells, he said.

Jensen concluded that independent of BMI, centralized fat distribution in the abdomen predicted larger fat cells, which appear most likely to cause metabolic abnormalities or dysfunction. Fat cell dysfunction predicted metabolic consequences (e.g., diabetes and hyperlipidemia). Furthermore, the evidence suggests that fasting hypertriglyceridemia could be an early sign of fat cell dysfunction in energy metabolism and its ability to take up triglycerides from the bloodstream after a meal and release fatty acids.

A HEALTH SYSTEM AND HEALTH SERVICES RESEARCH PERSPECTIVE ON THE USE OF BMI TO DIAGNOSE AND TREAT OBESITY

David Arterburn, senior investigator at the Kaiser Permanente Washington Health Research Institute and affiliate professor in the Department of Medicine at the University of Washington, was the second speaker; he discussed the practical implications to finance and deliver health care using BMI as a quality measure and the cost implications for alternatives.

Arterburn began by providing some context for BMI in health care. He introduced the National Committee for Quality Assurance (NCQA), which created the Adult BMI Assessment as a performance measure of U.S. adults that had an outpatient visit and who had their BMI documented (NCQA, 2023). In 2009, BMI was documented in 40 percent of health insurance plans and outpatient visitors' health records, and by 2019, that was over 80 percent of outpatient visits. However, in 2020, NCQA discontinued this because the electronic health record (EHR) automatically calculated BMI, and its performance was not measured alongside lifestyle counseling or other interventions.

Arterburn noted that in 2009, a BMI percentile measure was released for overweight and obesity in children and adolescents. One-third of children's EHRs included a BMI percentile, which jumped to over two-thirds of EHRs from 2009 to 2021, a considerable increase, he said.

As a standard measure in EHRs, BMI directs insurance coverage for obesity interventions, so Arterburn identified financial implications in health care. He pointed to a study of a nationally representative sample of adults from 2011 to 2016 (Ward et al., 2021). The results showed that a BMI of 18.5–24.9 kg/m^2 was associated with the lowest estimated expenditures and total health care costs and that costs increased for men and women with a BMI ≥ 35 kg/m^2. Furthermore, across BMI categories, women had slightly higher costs than men (see Figure 4-1).

In the same study, Arterburn detailed, BMI percentile or BMI z-scores in children and adolescents and the estimated total health care costs were steady across most BMI percentiles, save for a sharp increase for a BMI ≥ 99th percentile (see Figure 4-2).

After inflation adjusting these numbers to 2023, Arterburn estimated that health care expenditures (Ward et al., 2021) in U.S. adults with a BMI of 30–34.9 kg/m^2 were $7,300 per person,[1] increasing to $9,300 with a

---

[1] 2023 costs inflation adjusted from 2015 estimates from Ward et al. (2021) using https://www.bls.gov/data/inflation_calculator.htm (accessed September 22, 2023).

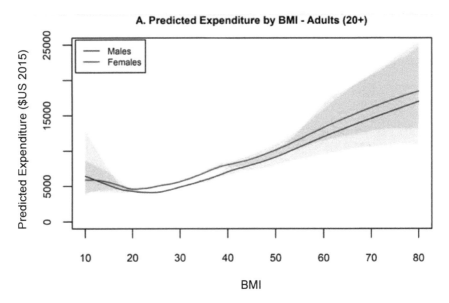

FIGURE 4-1 U.S. Medical Expenditure Panel Survey 2011–2016: Predicted expenditure by BMI in adults ages 20 and over.
NOTE: BMI = body mass index.
SOURCES: Presented by David Arterburn, April 4, 2023. Ward et al. (2021). Reprinted with permission.

BMI >35 kg/m². The estimated cost was 26 and 43 percent higher for a BMI over 30 kg/m² or over 35 kg/m², respectively, compared to the normal range (18.5–24.9 kg/m²). In 2023, Arterburn reported, 41 percent of Kaiser Permanente Washington region's health care system patients had a BMI of over 30 kg/m², which accounted for 50 percent of its health care costs.

Arterburn shifted to alternative measures for visceral fat and their costs and limitations. He admitted that waist circumference and digital anthropometrics are cost effective and possible in the clinical setting. However, the drawbacks are that staff must be trained, patients and staff often find the waist circumference uncomfortable to perform, and additional time is required. Referring to cost estimates from the *Healthcare Bluebook* (2022), a hypothetical laboratory test to improve the diagnosis of obesity could cost as much as $100 per test, but no viable option exists. He agreed with other presenters that dual X-ray absorptiometry (DEXA) is an accurate measure of visceral adiposity but also expensive, about $200 per test. A computerized tomography (CT) scan of the abdomen and magnetic resonance imaging are better measures of visceral adiposity and even more expensive, estimated at $750 and $1,250 per test, respectively.

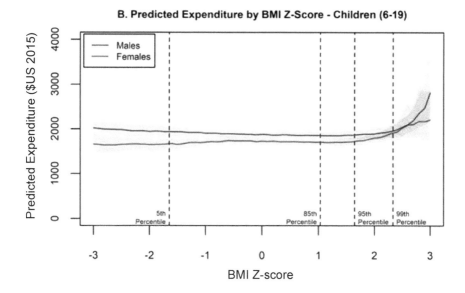

FIGURE 4-2 U.S. Medical Expenditure Panel Survey 2011–2016: Predicted expenditure by BMI z-score in children ages 6–19.
NOTE: BMI = body mass index.
SOURCES: Presented by David Arterburn, April 4, 2023. Ward et al. (2021). Reprinted with permission.

Arterburn described estimates for the Kaiser Permanente health care system with alternative measures for visceral fat in the clinical setting. He indicated that implementing these in a health care system would lead to a dramatic increase in costs. If screened annually in adults with a BMI of 30-34.9 kg/m², the estimated costs to the health system would be: $150 million per year for laboratory measures, $300 million per year for whole body DEXA, $1.13 billion per year for abdominal CT, and $1.88 billion per year for MRI. Although the cost for obtaining anthropometrics is listed as $0, staff training and time would be considerable.

Arterburn also described the financial implications of obesity treatment. Treatment guidelines recommend comprehensive lifestyle interventions for people with a BMI ≥30 or ≥25 kg/m² with comorbidities (Jensen et al., 2013). Based on these comorbidities, he estimated that up to 65 percent of U.S. adults could be eligible (unpublished estimates); 50–55 percent with a BMI ≥30 kg/m² or ≥27 kg/m² with comorbidities would be eligible for pharmacotherapy with a lifestyle intervention, and up to 30 percent could be eligible for metabolic surgery based on the American Society of

Metabolic and Bariatric Surgery updated guidelines, which includes patients with a BMI ≥35 kg/m^2 regardless of comorbidities, adults with a BMI of 30–34.9 kg/m^2 and a pre-existing metabolic disease, and an adjusted BMI cutoff (≥27.5 kg/m^2) for Asian Americans with an increased health risk (Eisenberg, 2022).

Arterburn reported on recent estimates that if 5 percent of adults with obesity in Medicare Part D received a prescription for semaglutide or phentermine and topiramate, it would cost $13 billion or $659 million (Baig et al., 2023), respectively.

Arterburn concluded that despite its limitations, BMI is more cost effective and efficient than alternatives. He acknowledged the heterogeneity for health risks in patients with a BMI <35 kg/m^2. From a practical, population health standpoint, Arterburn suggested narrowing the criteria for those who will benefit most from treatment instead of broadening them with uncertain benefit. He suggested that additional measures for adipose tissue distribution could help identify those who are at greatest risk for health complications and would benefit most from weight loss.

Arterburn concluded by posing questions when considering tests beyond BMI. Is the test supported by strong scientific evidence? Can it identify people at greater risk of adiposity-related disease? Is it acceptable to patients and providers? Are clinicians effective at administering it? What does it cost? Is a clinical study of treatments (e.g., lifestyle, pharmacotherapy, surgery) needed to test the safety and efficacy and cost effectiveness for new subpopulations identified by it?

OCCUPATIONAL HEALTH AND SAFETY LENS ON BMI

Alberto Caban-Martinez, a board-certified physician-scientist, associate professor of public health sciences, and deputy director of the M.D.–M.P.H. Program at the University of Miami, presented his perspective on the use of BMI for occupational health and safety. He opened by challenging the audience to consider how the work environment could support body weight management in the U.S. worker population, which accounts for 166 million of 334 million documented and undocumented people.

Caban-Martinez asserted that work is a social determinant of health; it establishes a person's income and economic stability and residence and neighborhood, which affects their access to schools and educational attainment, the availability of healthy and nutritious foods, and, of course, access to health insurance and health care.

Using data from the National Health Interview Survey, Caban-Martinez highlighted trends and the prevalence of obesity in the U.S. workforce from 1986 to 2002 (Caban et al., 2005). The results of his study showed that

Black men and women had a higher BMI rate than White men and women or others in the workforce (Caban et al., 2005).

Examining the data across occupational groups also showed differences in obesity prevalence. Police and firefighters exhibited a 2 percent increase, and blue-collar jobs, such as construction laborers, also had a 1.8 percent increase. Personal service occupations in skin care, hair care, animal care, and funeral service, farm workers, and other agricultural workers, exhibited a decrease, he said.

Caban-Martinez highlighted that women employed in motor vehicle occupations exhibited a 6 percent increase in obesity prevalence, and women in professional specialty occupations had a 2 percent increase. The prevalence among women employed as secretaries, stenographers, and precision production occupations decreased by ≤1 percent.

In 2014, Caban-Martinez shared, an updated paper examined occupations with the highest and lowest obesity prevalence. Employees in motor vehicle operation, construction and related work, law enforcement, and nursing, psychiatric, and home health aide had the highest prevalence; employees in health diagnosing, military, art and design work, and postsecondary school had the lowest (Gu et al., 2014).

Caban-Martinez provided some historical context, highlighting the evolution of the U.S. economy from industry to service-focused economy. In the 1940s, it was labor intensive, with its strengths in manufacturing, agriculture, and mining (Georgetown University Center on Education and the Workforce, 2018). From 1940 through 2016, manufacturing jobs declined significantly, and the U.S. economy shifted toward the service information sector, with greater employment opportunities in administration, educational services, financial activities, and health services (Georgetown University Center on Education and the Workforce, 2018). According to Caban-Martinez, this shift significantly impacted physical activity at work.

Caban-Martinez continued by sharing a recent study of U.S. workers aged 25–74 surveyed before, during, and after the COVID-19 lockdown that found that working from home was correlated with decreased physical activity (Streeter et al., 2021). Furthermore, fully remote workers were likely to spend more time sitting and less time exercising compared to those working partially from home and partially at their place of employment.

Looking at studies of obesity in firefighters in different geographical areas, Caban-Martinez discussed the potential challenges posed in the fire and rescue response. He presented a study with New York firefighters that found that 52 percent had obesity (Smith et al., 2012), compared to about 30 percent in Texas, Florida, and Missouri (Clark et al., 2002; Kling et al., 2020; Poston et al., 2011). Another study looked at a national sample of male firefighters and found that about 30 percent had obesity (Wilkinson et al., 2014). Caban-Martinez shared his research on the physical activity of fire and rescue responders using wearable devices and actigraphy while at the station and during rescue operations. When self-reporting, firefighters often mischaracterized their level of physical activity when compared to the actigraphy; firefighters who had obesity were the most inconsistent in their level of physical activity.

Caban-Martinez's research team also piloted a walking meeting to understand if it could reduce sedentary behavior in the office setting; a protocol was implemented and evaluated for its feasibility and acceptability in teams of fewer than six people. Workers wore actigraphy devices for 3 consecutive weeks. A baseline was established and followed to capture physical activity via the protocol. The findings indicated that, weather permitting, the meetings were largely accepted and increased the levels of moderate and very vigorous physical activity.

Caban-Martinez ended by highlighting opportunities to use the work environment to reduce sedentary behavior and improve body weight management, particularly in occupations with a demonstrated increase in obesity. He urged the audience to consider opportunities to work with employers, their employees, and the work environment to reduce sedentary behavior and support healthy body weight management through physical activity (Kling et al., 2016).

BMI OUTSIDE THE CLINIC: THE PATIENT PERSPECTIVE

Faith Anne Heeren, Ph.D. candidate at the University of Florida and founder and president of Outreach, Community, Engagement, Advocacy, Non-Discriminatory Support (OCEANS), a nonprofit advocacy group for adolescents with obesity, provided her perspectives and patient experience as a person living with obesity (OCEANS, 2023).

Heeren recounted that her weight trended in the 99th percentile from an early age. Her mother was concerned about her health and sought advice from health care providers. However, she found that their guidance was generally unhelpful (e.g., do not serve cookies for dinner) and not actionable or evidence based.

Despite her mother's efforts to serve her natural and sugar-free foods, Heeren continued, she gained weight through childhood and adolescence, developing hypertension and insulin resistance. Through online research, Heeren's mother discovered the Healthy Lifestyles program at Duke University that offered bariatric surgery for teenagers. Heeren decided to have bariatric surgery and attended monthly visits with Duke's multidisciplinary team in preparation.

Heeren immediately felt the physical and mental health benefits of surgery. Her insulin resistance and high blood pressure resolved and did not return. She had surgery in early summer before her junior year of high school, and by early fall, she had more energy and successfully earned a place on the varsity tennis team. Her confidence grew, and she began living a relatively carefree teenage life, shopping for prom dresses with friends, and participating in Senior Skip Day by walking limitlessly at the zoo. Her confidence was sustained in college, walking to classes on the UNC Chapel Hill campus, running 5K races, playing intramural sports, and participating in fitness classes at the student recreation center with friends. Heeren also started OCEANS to advocate for and offer support groups to adolescents living with obesity and undergoing treatment interventions.

Later in life, during graduate school and the COVID-19 lockdown, personal and family hardships and stress led to significant weight gain. She was challenged to complete activities of daily living without excessive fatigue and hip pain. In early 2023, she began to participate in an evidence-based behavioral weight-management program. After a month and a half, she lost weight, met with her provider to discuss anti-obesity medication, and had bloodwork that revealed additional health concerns. In February 2023, Heeren added topiramate. She achieved clinically significant weight loss and described less joint pain and more energy and confidence to continue monitoring her health and bloodwork. However, her health insurance refused to cover her weight-management services, so her plan is compromised and uncertain: "I have been on every side of the patient journey. I have had information and access to treatment, and now, I have information and am limited in my choices moving forward with treatment."

PANEL AND AUDIENCE DISCUSSION

Butsch led a moderated panel. The audience asked Jensen, Arterburn, Caban-Martinez, and Heeren about the effect of excess weight on the musculoskeletal system; utilization rates for obesity treatments and the impact on health care costs; costs for diabetes screening and medications to treat metabolic-related diseases; diversity and inclusion in walking meetings; measuring adipocytes in the clinical setting; and identifying adipocyte density through an ultrasound.

Impact of Excess Weight on the Musculoskeletal System
Beyond Cardiometabolic Health

An audience member opened the discussion with an appreciative comment for Heeren's presentation and emphasized the importance of learning about her increase in energy and decrease in joint pain with her weight loss. More attention is typically given to obesity and cardiometabolic health and less to the pressure on the musculoskeletal system or the mechanical implications of obesity, although they are clearly significant.

Caban-Martinez added that joint pain and lack of energy are important considerations, particularly for occupational health and safety; individuals who have obesity and work in manual labor, handling materials and staying in constant motion, often experience lower back and neck pain, with a load placed on the axial skeleton. Heeran's presentation on her quality of life and impact of weight on her musculoskeletal system emphasized that the same experience was common among people with obesity or excess body weight.

Real-World Utilization Rates for Bariatric Surgery Through Kaiser Permanente

Referring to Arterburn's presentation on using BMI or alternative measures to direct obesity treatment, a participant asked about data from Kaiser Permanente on the utilization rates for bariatric surgery. Arterburn responded that annually, 1–2 percent of members are eligible for and undergo it. However, the treatment guidelines encourage broader use; the cost estimate he presented was in response to these guidelines.

Data Availability on the Impact of Treatment on Health Care Costs

An audience member asked Arterburn about the increased cost of treating obesity and the medical care costs in his presentation. Are data available on the impact of different treatments on costs? Arterburn responded that data are not readily available, with a need for more research, including randomized trials, and long-term longitudinal studies to evaluate the impact of treatments on health care use and costs to evaluate their impact. He suggested that research could focus on patients with higher adiposity-related risks with measures to help identify subpopulations most likely to benefit from metabolic or mechanical treatments.

Diversity and Inclusion for People with Disabilities for Walking Meetings

An audience member commented on Caban-Martinez's presentation and cited examples of people with disabilities and cultural aspects of women's hair that may cause discomfort walking in a humid environment. They asked how issues of diversity and inclusion for people with visible and invisible disabilities are considered when promoting physical activity and exertion in the workplace, such as walking meetings. Caban-Martinez responded that only some work groups or offices can and should attend walking meetings. He emphasized the need for discussion about the capabilities, limitations, and concerns of potential participants when the meetings are proposed. Considerations can range from footwear and activewear to issues of interruption, all of which should be discussed beforehand.

Cost of Diabetes Screening and Medications

An online participant inquired about the cost of a routine diabetes screening test. Arterburn responded that a hemoglobin A1C test (HbA1C) costs much less than $100 per test. The current recommendation for diabetes screening is to screen most or all people with a BMI of over 30 kg/m^2 and those with a BMI over 25 kg/m^2 with another metabolic-related health condition to help identify people with diabetes or prediabetes (to prevent the progression to diabetes).

Butsch followed up, inquiring about the costs of antihypertensives or cholesterol medications. Arterburn said that pharmacotherapies for different health conditions vary widely in cost and their impact on weight and metabolic health but noted a need for long-term data on the effects of obesity medications on reducing the incidence of cardiometabolic disease or mortality.

Antihypertensives and cholesterol medications show reductions in cardiovascular events and mortality when tested in long-term randomized controlled trials, which supports their cost, said Arterburn. He pointed out the wide variation in their costs. Pharmacotherapy for type 2 diabetes, which can include the glucagon-like peptide 1 (GLP-1) receptor agonists and sodium–glucose cotransporter 2 (SGLT2) inhibitors that lower glucose, are expensive but increasingly proposed in the clinical guidelines. The cost of care for type 2 diabetes is rapidly escalating.

Measuring Adipocytes in the Clinical Setting

A participant commented that Jensen's presentation highlighted the size of adipocytes as predictive of metabolic health. How can the size of fat cells be measured and integrated into clinical settings? Jensen acknowledged the challenge and suggested that, ideally, providers could administer mini-liposuction or biopsy fat cells to determine their size, but this is unrealistic. Long term, he said, the goal is to have information available for providers to discern fat cell size, perhaps using fat distribution, sex, and age, without invasive procedures at regular appointments. However, fat cell size is irrelevant to the strain caused by excess weight on the musculoskeletal system.

Non-Health Care Professionals Communicating Technical Health Information to Students, Parents, and Workers

Butsch turned to BMI in school, asking Heeren about her experience and professional opinion. How is BMI used in that setting? Is it a surrogate marker? Heeren responded that in some school districts, parents receive a BMI report card for their child(ren). The problem, she said, is that parents do not always know how to interpret BMI or have access to evidence-based care to help guide what actions to take. So, she asked, what is the point of sharing BMI?

Caban-Martinez added that an objective from his study with firefighters with excess weight is to identify the most important technical, medical, and laboratory information and figure out how to optimally communicate with the participant.

Ultrasound Techniques to Identify the Density of Adipose Tissue

An audience member had a final question for Jensen. Could an ultrasound detect a difference in the density of adipose tissue with small versus large fat cells? Jensen responded that it is possible with new ultrasound techniques that have extremely high resolution; with ultrasound, researchers could identify fibrosis, vasculature, and characteristics of adipocytes. However, it is expensive, and acquiring funding for studies with it would be an obstacle.

5

Looking Ahead

The fourth and final session was moderated by Nico Pronk. He introduced the three panelists, whose presentations focused on an equity approach to address weight stigma, measuring success in obesity treatment, and the path forward for clinically assessing patients for obesity. He then led a panel and audience discussion.

Pronk reminded participants of the paradoxes surrounding body mass index (BMI) and obesity. Obesity diagnosed with BMI leads to broadly characterizing an endemic health problem that is socially and financially impervious. Pronk recalled that despite excess weight and elevated BMI, some people are metabolically healthy and show no limitations in activities of daily living. Yet, at the same time, the evidence clearly shows that obesity is associated with distinct pathophysiological alterations of tissues and organs, clinical signs, and symptoms, increasing the risk of secondary complications and multimorbidity. Obesity, defined as a disease, also justifies the need for access to medical treatment and care and may reduce weight-related bias and stigma.

Based on Stacy Wright and Faith Anne Heeren's presentations about their lived experiences, clinicians critically need to frame obesity and related measurements in the context of a patient's experience and focus on health risks, not weight. The challenge is to move beyond the relationship of BMI in defining obesity and its diagnosis, social and clinical implications, and patient experience.

AN EQUITY FRAMEWORK APPROACH
TO CHART NEEDED ACTION

The first presenter was S. Bryn Austin, who shared that her presentation would focus on weight stigma and discrimination using Shiriki Kumanyika's *Framework for Increasing Equity Impact in Obesity Prevention* (Kumanyika, 2017), which is designed to guide interventions to reduce disadvantage and improve equity. She began by presenting a definition of health equity:

> Health equity means everyone has a fair and just opportunity to be as healthy as possible. This requires removing obstacles to health, such as poverty, discrimination, and their consequences, including powerlessness and a lack of access to good jobs with fair pay, quality education, housing, safe environments, and health care. (Braveman et al., 2017)

Austin explained she used the upper right quadrant of the framework to focus on policy and systems change interventions for people living in large bodies (Kumanyika, 2017, 2019) (see Figure 5-1). She discussed two

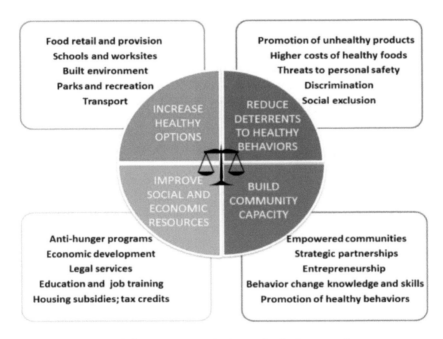

FIGURE 5-1 Framework for increasing equity impact in obesity prevention.
SOURCES: Presented by S. Bryn Austin, April 4, 2023. Kumanyika (2017). Reprinted with permission.

approaches to address equity issues and mitigate weight stigma and discrimination: legal action and eliminating barriers to care.

Austin presented background and evidence to demonstrate the severity of weight stigma and discrimination and the threats to personal safety for people living in larger bodies. She shared research documenting social exclusion and isolation, such as inaccessible public settings, and a myriad of attacks, including assumptions of negative characteristics, work-related discrimination associated with lower earnings, a lower probability for professional and educational advancement, a greater likelihood of being fired, and lower ratings by school teachers and college admissions professionals.

Austin detailed how these inequities significantly impact mental well-being and physical health, with a greater risk for depression, anxiety, eating disorders, and physiological stress and harmful physiological effects, such as the allostatic load or "wear and tear on the body" in response to discrimination.

Austin called out the widespread and legal weight discrimination in the United States, which is an obstacle to basic rights and health for people living in larger bodies (UConn Rudd Center for Food Policy and Health, 2017). She estimated that approximately 96 percent of people residing in the United States are in areas with no legal protection from weight discrimination.

Widening the scope to a macro level, Austin emphasized the societal and economic consequences of weight discrimination. Her research group, the Strategic Training Initiative for the Prevention of Eating Disorders (STRIPED), along with Deloitte Access Economics and Dove, authored a collaborative report on the social and economic cost of weight discrimination in U.S. society (Deloitte Access Economics, Dove, and STRIPED, 2022) that estimated that weight discrimination leads to an annual recurring cost of about $200 billion in the health system with productivity loss, wage loss, and employment loss.

Austin suggested banning weight discrimination to address the equity issue of discrimination and social exclusion. She pointed to a policy brief:

> Without laws to prohibit weight discrimination, people will continue to be unfairly fired, suspended, or demoted because of their weight, even if they demonstrate good job performance and even if body weight is unrelated to their job responsibilities. (UConn Rudd Center for Food Policy and Health, 2017)

Austin acknowledged the progress in passing antidiscrimination laws in Michigan and Washington state to protect people living in larger bodies (see Figure 5-2). She also highlighted that in the Massachusetts state legislature, Senator Rebecca L. Rausch and Representative Tram T. Nguyen have introduced legislation that prohibits discrimination against body size.

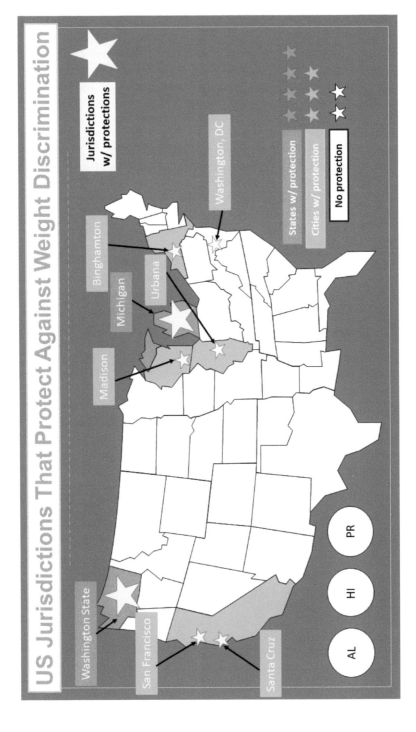

FIGURE 5-2 U.S. jurisdictions that protect against weight discrimination.
SOURCE: Presented by S. Bryn Austin, April 4, 2023. Reprinted with permission.

Austin continued by offering a second approach to address inequity and threats to personal safety from discriminatory practices affecting people living in larger bodies by expanding access to health care and eliminating barriers. The primary challenge, she admitted, will be to determine and agree on the barriers and strategies to remove them. One example of a barrier, Austin said, is the universal routine of weighing and BMI surveillance. She asked audience members to consider if universal weighing is a barrier to care. She noted that measurement of weight and BMI are ubiquitous in society, including in health care, online, in digital apps, at school, at work, and in athletics (Alberga et al., 2019; Austin and Richmond, 2022; Phelan et al., 2015; Richmond et al., 2021).

Austin suggested applying a strengths, weaknesses, opportunities, threats (SWOT) analysis to the idea of universal weighing or BMI surveillance. It is meant to systematically assess factors that may be helpful or harmful to a project and undermine or promote its success (AHRQ, 2021; Blayney, 2008; Minnesota Department of Health, 2021). Referring to universal weighing and BMI surveillance, she reminded participants that BMI is a poor health indicator and is used to justify persistent discrimination against people living in large bodies and disproportionately, minority communities.

Austin detailed the SWOT of universal weighing. The strengths include dosing medications, child health care and tracking their growth, and targeting efforts to improve public health and equity. She outlined opportunities that include being alerted to the impacts of interventions, societal trends, and inequities. However, she said, it also has clear weaknesses. Specifically, BMI is an unreliable proxy for individual health. Last, threats include widespread weight stigma that can cause a person to experience shame, avoid clinicians, and have poor health as a function of fewer health care visits and monitoring.

Austin urged the audience to consider where, how, and why routine weighing should be required or encouraged. How might practices disproportionately burden BIPOC (Black, Indigenous, and People of Color), low-income, and other minoritized communities receiving care through public systems? Austin advocated for clinicians to build relationships with their patients prior to discussing weight and concluded her talk with a quote from a physician in Washington, DC:

> I delay weighing new patients so I can make sure doing so would not cause harm, like in the case of clients with eating disorders or a history of body shame.

OBESITY TREATMENT:
HOW TO MEASURE SUCCESS FOR PUBLIC HEALTH

Craig M. Hales, clinical reviewer for the U.S. Food and Drug Administration Division of Diabetes, Lipid Disorders, and Obesity (serving in a personal capacity), was the second presenter. Hales emphasized that despite effective treatments available for obesity, it is not yet clear how to measure success for public health, as is the case for other chronic conditions.

Hales gave the example of hypertension. The goal of diagnosis and treatment is a specific blood pressure target, which is referred to as "controlled hypertension." With hypercholesterolemia, the goal is maximal atherosclerotic cardiovascular disease (ASCVD) risk reduction. For diabetes, the goal is a specific glycemic target. However, obesity has the unresolved question of how to define the goal of treatment.

Hales then reviewed four clinical guidelines for treating obesity. He began with the algorithm from the 2013 recommendations from American Heart Association/American College of Cardiology/The Obesity Society, which defines successful treatment as weight loss ≥5 percent, sufficient improvement in health targets as determined by the patient and clinician, and weight loss maintenance (Jensen et al., 2013). The Obesity Medicine Association's overall management goals for adults are to improve health, quality of life, and body weight, stating that 5–10 percent weight loss may improve metabolic disease (Tondt et al., 2023). He elaborated on the Endocrine Society's clinical guidelines on the pharmacological management of obesity, which mention ameliorating comorbidities and amplifying adherence to behavior changes, which may improve physical functioning and allow for greater physical activity (Apovian et al., 2015). For the pediatric population, the American Academy of Pediatrics (AAP) clinical practice guidelines indicate that a key is to monitor and treat comorbidities concurrently (Hampl et al., 2023). Furthermore, Hales added, AAP details the need for long-term data to establish weight loss and cardiovascular improvements impacting health into adulthood.

Hales moved on to discuss Healthy People 2030, which is a data-driven set of national objectives based on clinical guidelines to improve health and well-being over 10 years. To monitor progress toward the goals, a public health surveillance metric derived from clinical guidelines is required, although the various guidelines have no consensus on how to define successful obesity treatment as they do for other chronic conditions.

Hales then examined the public health surveillance metrics in Healthy People 2030 for other chronic conditions (Healthy People 2030, n.d.). For hypertension, an objective is to reduce the proportion of adults with high blood pressure, defined as systolic ≥130 mmHg or diastolic ≥80 mmHg, or taking an antihypertensive medication. Another objective is to increase the rate of blood pressure control for adults, which is defined as a systolic blood pressure <130 mmHg and diastolic blood pressure <80 mmHg. For hypercholesterolemia, Hales noted two objectives in adults: (1) reduce mean total blood cholesterol level in the population and (2) increase the rate of treatment among adults for whom a statin is recommended. For diabetes, the objectives are to (1) reduce the number of cases diagnosed annually and (2) reduce the proportion of adults with diabetes who have a hemoglobin A1c >9 percent.

However, in reviewing the Healthy People 2030 for overweight and obesity, Hales noted that the overall goal is to reduce both by helping people eat healthy and become physically active. He detailed three objectives: reduce the proportion of children and adolescents with obesity, reduce the proportion of adults with obesity, and increase the proportion of health care visits by adults with obesity that include counseling on weight loss, nutrition, or physical activity. The third objective addresses treatment but is a process measure and does not capture any health outcome that reflects successful management. For example, someone might be treated successfully and become metabolically healthy, but their BMI, as captured by public health surveillance, would categorize them simply as having obesity.

LOOKING AHEAD: CLINICAL ASSESSMENT OF OBESITY

Michael Knight was the last presenter. He provided a clinical perspective on defining obesity as a multifactorial disease. He opened by noting its many definitions, such as the following:

> A chronic, relapsing, multifactorial, neurobehavioral disease wherein an increase in body fat promotes adipose tissue dysfunction and abnormal fat mass physical forces, resulting in adverse metabolic, biomechanical, and psychosocial health consequences. (Obesity Medicine Association, 2017)

Knight shared that his patients often seek medical care for weight management. However, they list reducing their BMI as their health goal. Knight emphasized that the key to identify their goals is building a relationship, building trust, and coming to a shared understanding.

After all, Knight reiterated, BMI does not reliably predict adiposity. Some of his patients have an elevated BMI and no excess adiposity; others refuse to discuss weight because no one in their family has ever aligned with the BMI number. Still others have a lower BMI and metabolic dysfunction, underscoring the importance of assessing the whole patient, by listening and learning about their experiences.

As a clinician, Knight focuses on improving health outcomes, longevity, quality of life, and years of life to identify individuals with the greatest risk for morbidity and mortality. He introduced the Edmonton Obesity Staging

System (EOSS) as a useful framework to prioritize and predict health risks. It comprehensively assesses an individual and ranks the severity of obesity based on a clinical assessment of weight-related health issues.

A clinical diagnosis, Knight underscored, is an assessment of the whole person. For example, he said, a patient with diabetes and an HbA1C of 7.1 percent and no other issues will receive different medical treatment for diabetes management than a patient with an HbA1C of 6.9 percent who recently had a stroke and a myocardial infarction. Knight stated that HbA1C is only a number, like BMI. Similarly in hyperlipidemia, clinicians assess the risk for ASCVD, whereas they used to work with patients to achieve an LDL cholesterol under 130 mg/dl.

Knight asserted that the challenge is that BMI cutoffs direct treatment options (e.g., medication, surgery) and insurance coverage and clinician reimbursement. The functional component of obesity, meaning mechanical issues, such as joint pain and fatigue, can be significant despite no single reliable functional measure. Knight summarized that if a clinician only reviews a patient's BMI, the link to their health risk is missing.

PANEL AND AUDIENCE DISCUSSION

Pronk began the panel discussion. The audience asked the panelists questions about weight stigma and discrimination in the clinical setting; measuring success of obesity treatment; conversations with patients about BMI and its limitations; and reframing BMI as a vital sign and how to discuss its purpose with patients.

Addressing Weight Stigma and Discrimination in the Clinic

Pronk began by commenting to Austin about her talk on weight stigma and discrimination and policy implications. What can scientists and clinicians do to address these issues? Austin responded that scientists could address weight stigma by refraining from weighing patients at every visit. She recommended that clinicians talk with their patients about their experience with weight stigma to build a relationship for open dialogue. Austin also suggested that scientists and clinicians could promote and amplify the national anti-stigma campaign by the Obesity Action Coalition (OAC, 2023). Scientists and clinicians can also provide testimony and expertise to policy makers and their staff for evidence-based policy, she said.

Measuring Success in Obesity Treatment

An audience member commented on Hales' experience in the clinic and in public health and asked for his opinion on a measure for the success of obesity treatments. Hales said that he did not have a definitive answer, but it was instructive to consider the measures of success for other chronic conditions. One of the Healthy People objectives for hypertension defines the condition not only by blood pressure measurement but by recognizing that an adult may have been successfully treated, which is also a relevant concept for obesity.

Patient–Provider Conversations About BMI and Its Limitations

Knight received a question about how clinicians and providers could approach the conversation with patients about BMI and its limitations. Knight offered that many patients do not understand what BMI indicates other than it is a number reported during every clinic visit. Health care professionals could begin a conversation by explaining the reason for calculating BMI, what it screens for, and why it is not a health outcome. Knight advocated for clinicians to provide a foundational knowledge for context, give patients the ability to learn about their conditions and progress, and empower them to set personal goals. He urged clinicians and providers to consider BMI as a vital sign, like blood pressure.

Destigmatizing BMI as a Vital Sign: Conversations with Patients About Its Purpose

An audience member and clinician responded to Knight's comment to destigmatize BMI and frame it as a vital sign. How can clinicians and providers do so? Austin responded by reminding participants that she is not a clinician. She noted that everyone is weighed immediately at medical centers for any condition and advocated for refraining from doing so unless necessary, because it causes some patients to avoid medical centers, and that clinicians establish a rapport with a patient before weighing them.

Knight added that many patients do not understand the need for a weigh-in at every doctor's visit. Patients report that BMI or weight is sometimes but not always mentioned. Still, at other times, he said, the doctor may passively comment on a patient's need to lose weight without offering actionable steps. In weight-management clinics, weighing in is not an issue because patients are seeking weight-related services. Knight advised that if clinicians measure BMI, they must have a plan to address it.

CLOSING REMARKS

Ihuoma Eneli began by recalling that the planning committee chose the topics of BMI and the definition of obesity because of special interest among the U.S. public, as highlighted by the media. In 2021, several articles appeared on the limitations of BMI, including one in the February issue of *Good Housekeeping* on "The Racist and Problematic History of Body Mass Index" and one in *The Washington Post* on "Why BMI Is a Flawed Health Standard, Especially for People of Color." Eneli added that the Lancet Diabetes and Endocrinology Commission on the Definition and Diagnosis of Clinical Obesity was formed to gain consensus after reviewing the evidence for BMI and its role in defining obesity from the scientific and lived-experience perspectives; the final report will have substantial implications for the field, domestically and internationally. Eneli also pointed to the AAP guideline (January 2023) that outlines key actions for clinicians to discuss BMI or BMI percentile as a screener for health with patients and their families and use BMI percentile to assess the patient for risk factors for other conditions.

Eneli recapped the workshop that explored the science of body composition and body fat distribution measures and focused on the strengths and limitations of BMI as a measure of adiposity and health. She highlighted that the speakers examined the utility of alternative measures to assess obesity, morbidity, and mortality and their practical implications on defining obesity in health care, public health, and the legal field for prevention and treatment.

Eneli noted the points of agreement among scientists and clinicians. BMI measures body size and not body health. It is a surrogate measure of body fat and a screening tool with some reliable strengths, she added. It is simple to calculate, inexpensive, noninvasive, and highly familiar to patients, providers, and the public. She also emphasized that BMI is a standardized and objective measure that correlates with body fat and tracks the growth of children and population trends. Eneli reasoned that because of its strengths, BMI guides treatment options and reimbursement from insurers and serves as an objective endpoint in clinical trials.

Eneli also pointed to several limitations of BMI, underscoring that it is not a direct measure of body fat and does not capture fat distribution. It does not distinguish between lean body mass and fat mass, and evidence is lacking to support the cutoffs to define obesity, all of which have implications for different population segments. She stated that the association between BMI and body fat varies by race, ethnicity, and age. Moreover, in patients who have undergone bariatric surgery, a change in BMI is not indicative of changes in body fat. She added that BMI does not measure fat cell size, a developing measure for dysfunction. These inconsistencies have led to patients misinterpreting BMI, which also happens in health care, by employers, and in public health. The downstream effect is its contribution to weight bias and stigma, which are key elements of discrimination that impact public health and quality of life.

Eneli continued that the evidence presented at the workshop revealed that adipose tissue distribution in the visceral or ectopic areas versus subcutaneous tissue may be more predictive of metabolic disease or unhealthy obesity than BMI. Furthermore, she said, a genetic predisposition determines fat distribution through human biology and hormones, which vary by race, ethnicity, and age and account for differences in obesity and comorbidities across groups. Accordingly, BMI and visceral fat are moderately correlated.

Eneli highlighted other research presented that demonstrated the correlation between the size of adipocytes or fat cells and their functional capabilities. Studies showed that the larger the adipocyte, the greater the risk for dysfunction and metabolic health consequences. She recalled the example of a patient with a BMI of 35 kg/m^2 and healthy lab results with low cholesterol and noted a moderate and insignificant correlation between BMI and the size of fat cells.

Eneli discussed the alternative measures to BMI, which are limited by their accuracy and cost. Digital anthropometry is more indicative of health, although clinical trials need to test its reliability. She noted that waist circumference is a better measure and predictor of health, but providers/patients are uncomfortable when administering/enduring the measurement. Dual X-ray absorptiometry is more accurate than BMI, but it is cost prohibitive.

Eneli referred to the outstanding questions, tensions, and opportunities for future research. What is the physiology and pathophysiology of adipose tissue, and how does it help to define obesity? Does the available evidence support the cutoffs? Given the limitations of BMI, she questioned whether it should be eliminated or used for specific purposes. How are BMI and alternative measures interpreted in the clinical setting, health care, and public health? What are the potential implications of the alternatives regarding weight bias and stigma, cost, and society? How do clinicians communicate about the physical and psychosocial health considerations with a high BMI in policy, public health, and health care?

Eneli concluded by affirming that health is not merely the absence of disease and that obesity is not only about cardiometabolic health. Obesity affects physical health, mental health, and quality of life. She encouraged participants to return for the second workshop of the series (June 2023) on novel approaches to improve communication about body composition, BMI, adiposity, and health across diverse groups and sectors and strategies to mitigate disinformation and misinformation and identify research gaps and potential next steps to advance the field in research, clinical practice, and public health policy.

6

Communicating How Obesity
Is Defined and Diagnosed

The first session of the June 2023 workshop featured three presentations highlighting the work of the Lancet Commission on the definition and diagnosis of clinical obesity, communicating about it using a disease staging system, and specifically the Edmonton Obesity Staging System (EOSS) in the adult and pediatric populations. A panel and audience discussion followed. Ihuoma Eneli welcomed participants to the second workshop.

Eneli provided background and informed the audience of the two-part series, exploring the science and measuring body composition, body fat distribution, and obesity. The first workshop (April 2023), she explained, reviewed the World Health Organization (WHO) definition of obesity, examined it as a condition of excess body fat that impairs health, and outlined the strengths and limitations of body mass index (BMI) as a surrogate measure of body fat. Eneli shared that the second workshop builds on the first, focusing on how to communicate with diverse groups and sectors about body composition, BMI, adiposity, and health. She outlined the session topics, including strategies for providers to communicate with patients on the diagnosis and definition of obesity, influence and effects of weight bias and stigma, ethics and challenges in communicating about the intersection of weight and health, and long-term strategies to inspire a cultural shift on perceptions of weight.

THE LANCET COMMISSION ON THE DEFINITION
AND DIAGNOSIS OF CLINICAL OBESITY

Francesco Rubino, chair of metabolic and bariatric surgery at the King's College London, was the first presenter. He began by underscoring that obesity is not universally accepted as a disease and is widely considered a condition of excess adiposity that indicates an increased risk for future disease. The concept of it as a disease is not well developed, despite various clinical guidelines for treatment and management and national public health targets.

In medicine, Rubino continued, conditions that increase a person's risk to develop a chronic disease also present an opportunity to define strategic and efficient targets for treatment. The clinical signs and symptoms for a disease can range from activities of daily living to organ dysfunction. He said that BMI is not a clinical parameter and does not measure excess adiposity or indicate tissue or organ function.

Consequently, Rubino said, the clinical signs and symptoms for obesity and treatment targets are poorly defined. The lack of a clear causal sequence becomes apparent when providers apply prevention strategies that are unsuitable for severe obesity, complications, or comorbidities. Rubino stated that treatment plans that do not work can lead patients to become vulnerable to predatory advertisements for weight loss fixes in popular media. He summarized that the loose definition for obesity as a health condition (or disease) reinforces misinformation and disinformation and promotes weight stigma.

To illustrate this point, Rubino shared his research that surveyed people about their beliefs on the cause of obesity across four countries (O'Keeffe et al., 2020). One question asked if it could be cured through lifestyle changes, such as diet and exercise; respondents who agreed also scored higher for fatphobia, meaning they held more stigmatizing views. According to Rubino, the most significant contributor to stigma is a lack of understanding of obesity as a disease, which is invariably reversible without pharmacotherapy or surgical intervention.

Rubino affirmed that the concept of obesity as a disease is one of the most controversial and polarizing issues in medicine. Physician opponents point to patients with excess adiposity who do not show clinical manifestations (e.g., limitations of daily activities), although it is a marginal segment of patients, he said.

Rubino emphasized that BMI was not designed or intended as a clinical measure of excess adiposity. In its original form, it was a population-level measure for the increased risk of mortality. He pointed to football players and boxers as an outlier group with a high BMI because of their muscle or lean body mass.

Rubino added that BMI does not measure clinical manifestations of obesity in tissue or organs. Furthermore, the BMI-related risk for diabetes or mortality varies across groups segmented by ethnicity, age, and gender. Consequently, BMI cannot accurately reflect the risk for complications or mortality across population segments.

To address these issues, Rubino introduced the Lancet Commission on Clinical Obesity, which is tasked with generating a consensus among a group of 60 experts on the mechanisms underlying clinical manifestations of obesity as a disease. According to Rubino, it is developing a consensus report to determine the definition and diagnostic criteria for clinical obesity.

Rubino noted the substantial barriers to gain consensus among commission experts. Historically, he said, obesity has been described as excess adiposity that presents a risk to health. The commission is grappling with the etiology of the disease, distinct pathophysiology, and clinical manifestations or illness. A condition of risk is not per se a disease, he said.

Rubino shared several questions the commission is considering. Does obesity have a clinical phenotype? What is an accurate measure of excess adiposity, and is it necessary to diagnose obesity? With additional anthropometric measures, will patients present with an illness or clinical manifestation? Although experts will continue to deliberate on these topics, Rubino claimed agreement that BMI is an insufficient measure for obesity.

Rubino summarized that, in obesity, anthropometrics and BMI do not measure organ dysfunction. In some diseases, such as diabetes, biomarkers are strongly associated with clinical manifestations. He affirmed that the only way to determine the expression of obesity is to focus on clinical manifestations and that the consensus report will have profound implications for clinical practice, public health, and weight stigma.

ADIPOSITY-BASED CHRONIC DISEASE AND THE COMPLICATIONS-CENTRIC APPROACH TO DISEASE STAGING AND MANAGEMENT

W. Timothy Garvey, professor of medicine at the Department of Nutrition Sciences at the University of Alabama at Birmingham, gave the second presentation, which focused on obesity or adiposity-based chronic disease (ABCD) and its management using a complications-centric approach.

Garvey began by providing a time line and progression for ABCD. He stated that obesity was first regarded as a disease in 2012 by the American Association of Clinical Endocrinology (AACE) in a position statement that outlined the three criteria required for a disease diagnosis from the American Medical Association (AMA). Garvey maintained that obesity is a disease because of (1) characteristic signs or symptoms (excess adiposity measured by BMI) that (2) results in cardiometabolic and biomechanical complications (harm or morbidity), and (3) impairs the normal function of some aspect of the body (dysregulation of body functions).

To further define obesity, Garvey said, the AACE held a Consensus Conference on Obesity in 2014 with multidisciplinary stakeholders from different sectors, including biomedical, government and regulatory, health care, research, and education. It aimed to discuss and agree on the definition of obesity, determine available options to manage it, identify therapeutic modalities and their cost, and pinpoint knowledge gaps and decide how to approach them.

Garvey recounted the primary issue that emerged was that a diagnosis exclusively based on anthropometric measures (BMI) was unreliable. The consensus was that these did not measure excess adiposity or indicate an impact on health, particularly across racial and ethnic groups. Consequently, reliable treatment and health care benefits could not be determined, and no actionable policy steps were identified. However, conference stakeholders agreed on two components for an accurate diagnosis: (1) a measure for excess adiposity; although BMI is imperfect, it is ingrained worldwide; and (2) a manifestation of severe complications, confirming morbidity and mortality (Garvey et al., 2014).

Two years later, the AACE Obesity Guidelines were released for obesity management using a complications-centric approach to care (Garvey et al., 2016). The goal was to treat the cardiometabolic, biomechanical, and quality of life complications that impaired health. He emphasized that the endpoint was not weight loss but preventing and treating complications.

Garvey detailed the three stages outlined in the guidelines. The algorithm included two diagnostic components: anthropometrics and clinical manifestation to guide treatment. Stage 0 represented an absence of complications. Stage 1 was characterized by mild to moderate complications and aimed to treat and prevent or limit complications with weight loss. Stage 2 included severe complications and involved pharmacotherapy and/ or surgery.

Garvey shared that in the 2016 AACE guidelines, risk was stratified using clinical stages, which are simple and intuitive for clinicians to use and cost effective because evidence-based therapy is expensive. Weight-loss therapy can prevent the progression from the clinical stages to end-stage manifestations, leading to risk for other diseases, and also treat end-stage manifestations, prevent the onset of other diseases, and limit polypharmacy.

Garvey moved on by explaining the three types of health complications from obesity (see Figure 6-1). The first is quality of life, which negatively impacts mental health (e.g., anxiety) and physical health (e.g., pain). The second is cardiometabolic, leading to poor metabolic and vascular outcomes, such as insulin resistance and prediabetes, metabolic syndrome, dyslipidemia, prehypertension, and hepatic steatosis. The third type is biochemical and a function of excess body fat over time.

Garvey recalled that shortly after the release of the guidelines, AACE and the American College of Endocrinology introduced a more precise and medically actionable diagnostic term to convey obesity as a disease and not just an elevated BMI (Mechanick et al., 2017):

Categories of Obesity Complications

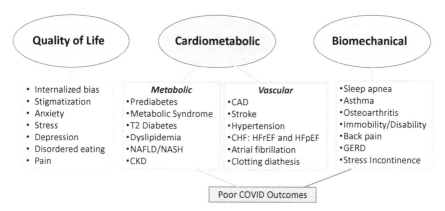

FIGURE 6-1 Categories of obesity complications.
NOTE: T2 = type 2; CAD = coronary artery disease; CHF = congestive heart failure; CKD = chronic kidney disease; GERD = gastroesophageal reflux disease; HFrEF = heart failure with reduced ejection fraction; HFpEF = heart failure with preserved ejection fraction; NAFLD/NASH = nonalcoholic fatty liver disease/nonalcoholic steato hepatitis.
SOURCE: Presented by W. Timothy Garvey, June 26, 2023. Reprinted with permission.

> Adiposity-Based Chronic Disease (ABCD) is a new diagnostic term for obesity that explicitly identifies a chronic disease, alludes to a precise pathophysiologic basis, and avoids the stigmata and confusion related to the differential use and multiple meanings of the term "obesity."

Abnormalities in the mass, distribution, and function of adipose tissue, a lifelong chronic disease, may lead to health complications, morbidity, and mortality.

Garvey discussed the Cardiometabolic Disease Staging System, for which he tested the efficacy by stratifying adults in the national CARDIA Cohort (Guo et al., 2014). Stage 0, he said, represents a metabolically healthy individual without any metabolic syndrome traits. Stage 1 denotes one or two metabolic syndrome risk factors. Stage 2 is characterized by impaired fasting glucose, impaired glucose tolerance, or metabolic syndrome. Stage 3 denotes two of three conditions or impaired fasting glucose, impaired glucose tolerance, or metabolic syndrome. Stage 4 indicates type 2 diabetes and/or cardiovascular disease. Garvey highlighted that people who met the criteria for prediabetes and metabolic syndrome (Stage 3) had a 40-fold increased risk for diabetes and all-cause and cardiovascular disease mortality compared to Stage 0.

According to Garvey, although these issues were paramount in the progress of diagnosing and treating obesity, the foremost issue is the International

Classification of Diseases, Tenth Revision (ICD-10)—it charts disease prevalence over time. Its code E66 is used for health care–related billing for treatment in the United States and several other countries. He pointed out that E66 indicates that the conditions are the result of excess calorie consumption, which is scientifically incorrect and medically unactionable. Garvey stressed that calorie counting would not track obesity treatment; it reinforces an inaccurate medical concept, promotes stigmatization, and limits public health.

Garvey then introduced an alternative ICD-10 coding that he and his colleague, Jeffrey I. Mechanick, proposed, which is scientifically accurate and medically actionable. The distinction between it and the current ICD-10 is that obesity is designated as a pathophysiological category without overt cause, caused by a genetic abnormality, or aggravated by other causes (e.g., endocrine, iatrogenic, disability) (Garvey and Mechanick, 2020).

Garvey explained that the B code signifies the BMI classification or a measure of the degree of adiposity. A C code identifies obesity-related complications bucketed into five categories with unique codes. A D code classifies the severity of the complication as mild, moderate, or severe. One example, Garvey offered, is sleep apnea, which would have a unique code. Severity criteria would use the apnea/hypopnea index: a score of <5 would be normal, a score of 5–30 would be mild to moderate, and a score of >30 would be severe.

Garvey concluded that the principles underlying the alternative ICD-10 coding and staging systems for ABCD are based on the presence, severity, and risk of related complications, and he urged their adoption to assist with decisions related to disease management.

EOSS FOR ADULTS AND PEDIATRICS

Geoff Ball, professor and associate chair of research in the Department of Pediatrics and the Alberta Health Services Chair in Obesity Research in the Faculty of Medicine and Dentistry at the University of Alberta, gave the third presentation. Ball continued the discussion on the value of staging in obesity by focusing on the EOSS and its application to the pediatric population (Sharma and Kushner, 2009).

Ball began by providing the background and overview of the EOSS, a clinical and functional staging system (Sharma and Kushner, 2009). It identifies the consequences of obesity with increasing severity by stage (0–4) and outlines relevant strategies for prevention and management (Sharma and Kushner, 2009).

Ball informed the audience that the EOSS was published in 2009 and aimed to be an accurate measure for obesity. A nationally representative sample of adults from the National Health and Nutrition Examination

Survey (NHANES) dataset were stratified by EOSS score, which demonstrated that the severity of health consequences increased with it but not with BMI as a stand-alone measure (Kuk et al., 2011; Padwal et al., 2011). The survival curves diverged when stratified by EOSS score but not by BMI class (see Figure 6-2). EOSS also differentiated between those with low and greater health risks, revealing the specificity of EOSS, he said.

Ball moved on to the Edmonton Obesity Staging System for Pediatrics (EOSS-P) that he and his colleagues developed (Hadjiyannakis et al., 2016).

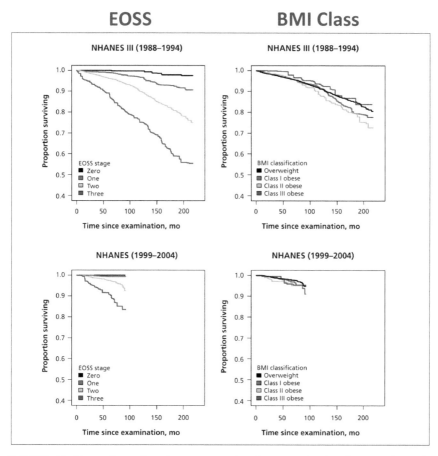

FIGURE 6-2 Comparison of staging system and anthropometric classification scheme for predicting all-cause mortality among people with overweight and obesity.
NOTE: BMI = body mass index; EOSS= Edmonton Obesity Staging System; NHANES = National Health and Nutrition Examination Survey.
SOURCES: Presented by Geoff Ball, June 26, 2023. Padwal et al. (2011). Reprinted with permission.

He shared four domains of health risk factors in the EOSS-P: mental, metabolic, mechanical, and social milieu. Ball explained that each of the domains is scored from 0 to 3, and the highest score in any domain is the EOSS-P score (also 0–3) (see Figure 6-3). He noted that in the pediatric population, anthropometrics reliably identified health risk using the EOSS-P across weight categories (Hadjiyannakis et al., 2019).

Ball elaborated that the EOSS-P provides a comprehensive health assessment of children's health. To illustrate how it works, he presented two case studies.

The first was a 12-year-old boy with severe obesity (see Figure 6-4). In each of the four domains, the boy scored 0, for an overall EOSS-P score of 0. Ball commented that it may be surprising for a boy with severe obesity to be in Stage 0. However, research has shown that approximately 10–15 percent of children who have severe obesity are in this category; they are typically younger and have less visceral or central adiposity. Ball pointed out that using an anthropometric measure, such as BMI, would tell a different, abbreviated story.

Ball introduced a second case study to demonstrate how the EOSS-P can differentiate health risk for children with the same BMI z-score (see Figure 6-5). Reviewing the scores in each of the four domains, mental

The 4Ms of EOSS-P

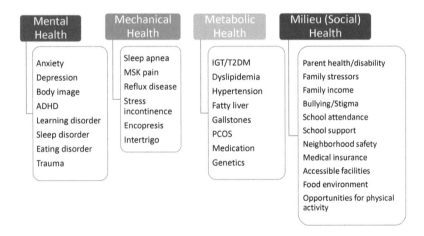

FIGURE 6-3 The 4Ms of EOSS-P.
NOTE: ADHD = attention-deficit/hyperactivity disorder; BMI = body mass index; EOSS-P = Edmonton Obesity Staging System for Pediatrics; IGT/T2DM = impaired glucose tolerance/type 2 diabetes mellitus; PCOS = polycystic ovary syndrome.
SOURCE: Presented by Geoff Ball, June 26, 2023. Reprinted with permission.

Case #1: 12-year-old boy with severe obesity (BMI z-score: 3.4)

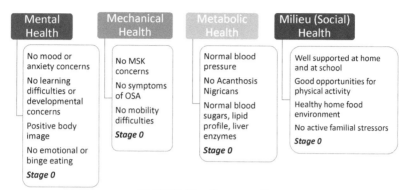

EOSS-P: Stage 0

FIGURE 6-4 Case #1: 12-year-old boy with severe obesity (BMI z-score: 3.4).
NOTE: BMI = body mass index; EOSS-P = Edmonton Obesity Staging System for Pediatrics;
MSK = musculoskeletal system; OSA = obstructive sleep apnea.
SOURCE: Presented by Geoff Ball, June 26, 2023. Reprinted with permission.

Case #2: 12-year-old boy with severe obesity (BMI z-score: 3.4)

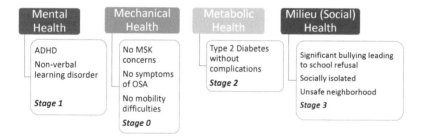

EOSS-P: Stage 3

FIGURE 6-5 Case #2: 12-year-old boy with severe obesity (BMI z-score: 3.4).
NOTE: ADHD = attention-deficit/hyperactivity disorder; BMI = body mass index; EOSS-P =
Edmonton Obesity Staging System for Pediatrics; MSK = musculoskeletal system.
SOURCE: Presented by Geoff Ball, June 26, 2023. Reprinted with permission.

health (1), mechanical (0), metabolic (2), and social milieu (3), generates an EOSS-P score of 3. The boy has ADHD and a nonverbal learning disorder (mental health), has type 2 diabetes without complications (metabolic), and is socially isolated in an unsafe neighborhood where he has experienced severe bullying (milieu). Ball reminded the audience that an anthropometric measure would be the same as in the first case study.

Ball highlighted an observational cohort study that examined the health risks of 850 boys in Canada and tested the association between the EOSS-P and the WHO BMI classification (Hadjiyannakis et al., 2019). The results showed that mental health concerns were most common of the four EOSS-P domains. Metabolic and mental health were equally distributed across BMI classes, and the social milieu and mechanical health challenges were more common in children with class III obesity. He also shared that BMI class underestimated disease burden in some children, overestimated it in others, and did not identify health risks. Ball ended by emphasizing that in the same study, the EOSS-P revealed health risks across weight categories.

PANEL AND AUDIENCE DISCUSSION

Scott Butsch led the audience and panel in a moderated discussion. Questions from the audience focused on the differences between the EOSS and EOSS-P; differences between the terms "obesity" and "ABCD"; communicating with patients about internalized weight bias; and the Lancet Commission's engagement with researchers in nutrition and social science.

Differences Between the EOSS and EOSS-P

Butsch asked the first question to Ball, who responded that the EOSS-P has fewer categories because obesity and its process do not manifest in children as they do in adults, such as a relatively low prevalence of type 2 diabetes, hypertension, and obesity-related conditions.

He also mentioned some subjectivity in the social milieu domain of the EOSS-P. The results depend on the instrument used, the person reporting symptoms or experiences, and whether the respondent is a parent or a child.

Developing tools for clinicians requires thinking about the end user and the ability to integrate into electronic health records (EHRs). Novel approaches must be easy, evidence based, and reliable.

Communicating with Patients About Internalized Weight Bias and the Biology of Weight Regulation

Butsch turned to Rubino's presentation on internalized weight bias among patients with overweight or obesity. How can clinicians communicate and bring this bias into a discussion with patients in a surgical clinic? Rubino said that internalized weight bias is clear in his practice and that patients are typically apologetic and feel they need to justify their bariatric surgery.

Patients seeking surgery for other problems, such as for the gallbladder, expect to be treated with respect and recognized as needing medical attention for a medical problem. They do not feel the need to justify their surgery. Medical professionals are partly responsible for internalized weight bias because of their focus on fixing obesity through lifestyle changes.

Rubino shared that when talking with bariatric surgery patients, he starts by explaining the biology of weight regulation and that patients cannot undo obesity at will, which normalizes the patient–provider relationship.

Garvey added that a recent AACE policy statement calls out internalized weight bias as a parameter for clinicians to assess in all patients. It must be identified like other health complications because it affects quality of life and the success of medical treatment, and it is an area for future study.

Differences Between Obesity-Related Terminology: ABCD Versus Cardiometabolic Disease

An audience member asked Garvey if ABCD is also a cardiometabolic disease. Furthermore, what is the difference between "complication" and "comorbidity in ABCD?" Garvey reiterated that obesity is not a cardiometabolic disease but that it has a complex interrelationship. Furthermore, he said, obesity is not required for cardiometabolic disease. Someone with ample lean body mass may have cardiometabolic disease if fat is distributed in their intra-abdominal area and they have inflammation and structural changes in their fat tissue. The reason that most patients who are diagnosed with cardiometabolic disease also have excess adiposity or obesity is that excess adiposity exacerbates it, and it can improve with weight loss.

Garvey noted that the Lancet Commission is addressing the term "complication." Rubino added that commission members have different opinions about comorbidities versus complications. According to Garvey, a comorbidity of obesity is a related complication, disease, or condition that occurs because of it. However, the commission report will distinguish between comorbidities and conditions, disorders, or diseases based on the pathophysiology of obesity.

EOSS for Adults Versus Children

The audience posed two more questions for Ball about the differences between EOSS-P and EOSS. Do the four domains apply only to the pediatric population (EOSS-P)? How is BMI incorporated into the adult EOSS? Ball reiterated that the four domains can stand alone and were designed to group multiple health indicators into one measure; some measures may be missing from the EOSS-P.

Garvey noted evidence that childhood obesity shortens the life span by 10 years and emphasized the seriousness of it. He asked how the staging in pediatrics relates to adult health?

Ball considered Garvey's concern as the reason for tracking EOSS-P scores over time. The scores have some predictive use but vary based on the person administering the EOSS-P. If obesity is a dysfunction of the weight regulatory system early in childhood, he explained, an adolescent may not have any complications of obesity, yet still have it.

Rubino added that regardless of the approach or staging, all three panelists agree that BMI cannot be a clinical parameter. The Lancet Commission is addressing the pediatric area of research in terms of how to define the illness of obesity.

Lancet Commission Engagement with Nutrition and Social Science Researchers

An audience member commented on the social and environmental impacts of obesity, asking whether the Lancet Commission is discussing it with nutrition and sociology researchers. According to Garvey, because obesity is linked to several other chronic conditions, such as diabetes, cardiovascular disease, and nonalcoholic fatty liver disease, the commission is consistently interacting and engaging with researchers at professional meetings, such as the American Diabetes Association.

7

Innovations in Communicating About Body Weight in the Clinic and Beyond

The second session, moderated by Craig Hales, was dedicated to innovations for providers to communicate with patients about body weight in the clinical setting and beyond. The first presentation focused on educating future clinicians about weight bias and stigma, followed by a presentation on speaking with patients about body positivity in a culture of obesity treatment and weight loss. Afterward, Hales facilitated an audience and panel discussion.

EDUCATING FUTURE CLINICIANS ABOUT WEIGHT BIAS AND STIGMA

Kofi Essel is a board-certified community pediatrician at Children's National Hospital, assistant professor of pediatrics and director of the School of Medicine and Health Sciences Culinary Medicine Program, Community/Urban Health Scholarly Concentration, and Clinical Public Health Summit on Obesity at George Washington University (GWU). Essel's presentation was on obesity stigma, its effects on medical and allied health care students, and strategies to reduce weight bias, stigma, and shame among students in universities.

Essel began by noting that faculty must recognize that medical students do not come into their training as blank slates and that it is necessary to be aware that their past lived experiences greatly influence their polarized perspectives on patients with obesity. Adding discussion of obesity stigma into a formal curriculum is critical, because if not, students absorb a hidden curriculum of cynicism seen in images and heard in comments from professors and providers that are engrained in clinical training.

Essel called out medical education, clinicians, and health care providers as all having played a role in amplifying weight bias and stigma. He pointed to Children's Healthcare of Atlanta, which spearheaded the social marketing campaign "Stop Sugarcoating It, Georgia," with images of children who have overweight and obesity on billboards. Although the campaign intended to bring awareness to the rising rates of obesity in children, it perpetuated weight stigma. According to Essel, campaigns such as this strategically and intentionally dehumanize, belittle, humiliate, and stigmatize people with overweight and obesity.

Essel highlighted research that has shown physicians describe patients who have overweight or obesity as noncompliant, lacking self-control, less healthy, less intelligent, and having lower self-esteem (Huizinga et al., 2010; Puhl and Heuer, 2009). When medical students learn of these reactions, they are shocked and assume it is not relevant to them because they will be different. Essel highlighted this as the opportune moment to expose students to their own biases and teach strategies to provide person-centered care and communicate about overweight and obesity with patients.

Essel and a team of faculty designed the Public Health Summit to teach medical students about how to engage obesity with tools of health equity and empathy. He described the almost 30 hours of curriculum to be a rare opportunity to educate them about the complexity of obesity and stigma and discuss these topics with peers and instructors. Shiriki Kumanyika's *Framework for Increasing Equity Impact in Obesity Prevention* (Kumanyika, 2017, 2019) guides the summit; medical students learn about the harmful effects of obesity stigma from people with lived experience and receive a population health perspective centering on health equity by working with local community-based organizations, state agencies, and numerous key stakeholders.

Essel noted that the summit was in its 8th year and has provided him and his colleagues an opportunity to create a formula and curriculum to train medical students on weight bias and stigma. Activities include the Harvard Implicit Association Test (IAT) on weight and a reflection exercise designed by Tom Sherman at Georgetown University on the students' experiences engaging patients with obesity. He emphasized the importance of anonymous responses to the reflection exercise, so that students are honest about their experiences without fear of judgment or retaliation.

Essel shared that most students have an implicit bias toward people living with large bodies. Unpublished data from the summit from 2018 to 2023 shows that over three-quarters of attendees preferred thinner body frames; 10 percent preferred larger body frames, and about 15 percent did not have a preference. Nationally, research shows the same trends of implicit bias against people with overweight and obesity among medical students (Miller et al., 2013).

When students are confronted with their bias, Essel continued, many are in denial, and skeptical of the IAT test and its results, and confused about the implications of the findings:

> I am skeptical of this [my] result. I found the test instructions rather confusing. Therefore, I do not necessarily believe that the IAT-weight is the best measure of a person's attitudes toward overweight people.

Essel highlighted other student responses, including the uncoupling of implicit versus explicit bias, meaning a student believes they have an innate ability to separate what they think about patients internally (conscious or subconscious) from how they treat patients. Students also reveal overt bias in response to their implicit bias:

> I do not think someone being obese means that they are bad people or less deserving of health care or other basic human rights. I do think it means that they do not really care about their health, or they are just less informed about health issues related to obesity, which does make me judge them a bit on that front. I think a little bit of stigma against obesity honestly would not be the worst thing. If anything, it would serve as an incentive for people to try and lose weight.

Essel described these perspectives as remnants from their formative years that can become integrated into their knowledge as medical students, amplified, and affect how they treat patients and their families later on when they become physicians.

Last, Essel said, some students react with rugged individualism (they were overweight and have lost weight). They view their weight loss as having gained control of their life and are confident and often condescending toward others, indicating that if they could lose weight, anyone can lose weight.

Essel offered 10 lessons learned from the summit that are relevant for all health care professionals (Alberga et al., 2016; Haqq et al., 2021; Kirk et al., 2020; MacInnis et al., 2020; Rubino et al., 2020). First, providers must increase their awareness of personal and collegial bias against obesity with tools such as the IAT-weight. Second, staff and colleagues must be trained to counteract bias against obesity using experiential learning and narratives from patients with obesity through their health care system or organizations such as the Obesity Action Coalition. Third, obesity must be recognized and taught as a complex, multisystem disease and not just a number on the scale. Essel agreed with other presenters that it is not always easily managed with lifestyle changes alone. Fourth, health care professionals must respect patient autonomy. Some do not want to lose weight or discuss weight at every visit. He said that the new craze around the "Please don't weigh me" cards is a response to health care not providing a safe space for patients and families, forcing them to take their dignity and humanity in their own hands. Sixth, he indicated that health should be taught as the primary goal, not cosmetic thinness or Western beauty standards. Weight is a contributing factor for many conditions and chronic diseases, but the role of physicians and allied health care professionals, he emphasized, is to support families in improving health, treat patients with dignity, and recognize their humanity. This sometimes will require strategies to directly support weight loss, but never should be viewed external to health. Seventh, an equitable health care environment must be created to accommodate and serve a range of patients with equipment that meet the needs of people with different body sizes. Eighth and ninth, he recommended that clinicians use people-first language and nonstigmatizing images of people with obesity. Tenth, he urged students and colleagues to take the pledge of the international joint statement to eliminate weight stigma (Rubino et al., 2020).

NAVIGATING DISCUSSIONS GRACEFULLY IN A BODY POSITIVITY VERSUS OBESITY TREATMENT WORLD

Robyn Pashby, a clinical health psychologist who specializes in the cognitive, behavioral, and emotional factors of health behavior change, was the second presenter focusing on body positivity and obesity treatment as two divergent yet overlapping styles of understanding.

As Sarah Tyrrell has said, "I was raised to believe fat was the worst thing a girl could be." Today's environment has a range of perspectives on weight, body image, and language. For example, some people practice body positivity, others subscribe to the concept of Health at Every Size,[1] and still others feel shame about their weight and self-advocate with the "don't weigh me" card that Essel mentioned. Providers must navigate these fundamentally different viewpoints when discussing health and obesity, Pashby said.

Pashby suggested that people may understand obesity without understanding how to talk about it. Professional organizations have made countless efforts to help define obesity but rarely offered an opportunity to understand ways to talk to people about it. One example was that individuals in the fields of science and medicine advocate for providers to use people-first language (e.g., "person with obesity") because a person is not their disease (see Figure 7-1). However, research shows that patients do not necessarily prefer this, favoring words such as "weight," "healthy weight," and "chubby" (Brown and Flint, 2021; Puhl, 2020; Puhl et al.,

---

[1] https://asdah.org/health-at-every-size-haes-approach (accessed September 15, 2023).

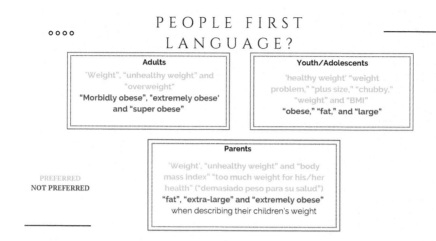

FIGURE 7-1 Examples of people first language.
SOURCES: Presented by Robyn Pashby, June 26, 2023 (data from Brown and Flint, 2021; Puhl, 2020; Puhl et al., 2022). Reprinted with permission.

2022). She emphasized that this example illustrates the need for clinicians and health care providers to continue listening and learning from patients.

Pashby turned to offering four concrete strategies to help bridge the gap between body positivity and obesity treatment in clinical practice and elsewhere. First, clinicians must understand the gap between body positivity and obesity treatment. According to Pashby, the conflict stems from the erroneous belief that body positivity promotes obesity. Pashby assured the audience that it is a movement for acceptance of all bodies regardless of their size, shape, skin tone, gender, physical abilities; it does not promote obesity.

Pashby reminded the audience that the U.S. weight-loss culture equates weight loss with aesthetics. For example, a recent social media advertisement promoted ways to "dress slim." Weight-loss culture is not about health, and a person experiencing internalized weight bias will still do so after they lose weight. Pashby affirmed that weight is not the issue with weight bias.

Second, Pashby challenged the audience to reconsider their assumptions about weight and weight loss and reflect on how it impacts their perspective of people with obesity. She suggested clinicians consider whether every patient wants to be thinner and whether body size is an indicator of nutrition knowledge and the effort to eat healthy and exercise.

The third strategy was for clinicians and providers to make "better" assumptions. Patients may or may not want to lose weight or be body positive. A person who is overweight may be very knowledgeable about taking care of themself and have put forth sustained and exhausting effort for their health. She encouraged providers to assume that patients can make health care decisions even if these are not aligned with the provider's clinical judgment and that their patients may feel alone, judged, and shamed, blame themselves, and have a strong need to please their provider. Consider the ramifications of a patient agreeing to lose 10 pounds between doctor's visits who does not or cannot achieve that, she said.

The fourth strategy is to learn and adopt trauma-informed care (Green et al., 2015). Assume a patient has experienced a traumatic stressor—not just adverse childhood events but also the traumatic stress of living in a larger body. She underlined that trauma-informed care is not trauma treatment. Rather, it accounts for the possibility that every patient may have a history of trauma exposure and forces clinicians to consider safety and transparency in the patient–provider relationship based on trustworthiness, collaboration, and cultural sensitivity.

Next, Pashby outlined steps providers can take to communicate and engage patients about a health concern for which they feel shame (e.g., bariatric surgery). She suggested that clinicians consider the context of an appointment and talk to patients about their thoughts and feelings and not just the outcomes. Providers need to consider the barriers to lifestyle changes and the tone of their voice, ask permission to speak about a given topic, and use trauma-informed care.

Pashby then presented three scenarios and example scripts for clinicians to use when communicating with patients about their health concerns.

In the first scenario (see Figure 7-2), Pashby described a patient who tells their clinician, "I want to lose 100 pounds." The starting point for responding is to consider their perspective. She suggested discussing their thoughts and feelings because these strongly impact behavior. Is the patient trying to beat their clinician to the punch? Do they assume the clinician will comment on their weight? Are they ashamed, frustrated, or exhausted? Are they worried about their health? What is the context of the appointment? If the patient is there for strep throat, how would they react to a pamphlet about bariatric surgery? She encouraged clinicians to imagine responding to the patient with "Let's build on what you are already doing to care for yourself."

Pashby presented a second scenario at an annual physical exam (see Figure 7-3). The clinician thinks the patient's health may be impacted by their weight. She recommended that they consider the patient's perspective and focus on their thoughts and feelings, not the outcome. Is the patient intentionally avoiding a discussion about their weight? Do they feel hopeless and stuck, or are they practicing body positivity or Health at Every Size? Are they in an active or recovery phase of an eating disorder? Imagine

WHAT TO SAY?

"Is it alright if we talk more about that? Can you tell me more about what you're thinking?"

"Your weight is bothering you. It is common for people to feel stuck and I am glad you are willing to talk to me. I am not here to judge, only to help."

"Let's build on what you are already doing to care for yourself. Working towards helping our bodies be and stay healthy is something we all have to do and I am happy to help you."

"If you are feeling stuck, let's identify some small, intermediate steps we can work towards together."

"Are you interested in learning more about medical treatments?"

"Weight is much more complicated than eat less, move more. I would like to help you get the support you need. Can I give you the name of someone who may be able to help more consistently than me?"

FIGURE 7-2 Sample script for Scenario 1.
SOURCE: Presented by Robyn Pashby, June 26, 2023. Reprinted with permission.

WHAT TO SAY?

"Would it be okay if we talk about your weight as part of your overall health today?"

"Could we talk about how you are feeling about your physical and mental health lately? Are there any health behaviors you'd like some support in changing? Almost everyone has something they are working on and I'd like to help."

"Are you wanting support to manage your weight? Weight isn't entirely in your control, and I am happy to work with you to make some small changes in areas you feel ready to change."

"So many factors contribute to overall health: stress, sleep, weight, social connections, mental health, and more. Your labs suggest that some of your health concerns may be better managed with some behavioral changes, but I know behavior change is hard. How can I help or support you as we work together towards improving your health?"

FIGURE 7-3 Sample script for Scenario 2.
SOURCE: Presented by Robyn Pashby, June 26, 2023. Reprinted with permission.

responding to the patient with "Would it be okay if we talk about your weight as part of your overall health today?"

The third scenario Pashby offered was at a pediatric appointment with parents about their child's weight (see Figure 7-4), which is complicated. Begin the conversation from a place of openness, safety, and transparency. She appealed for clinicians to consider changes for the family when thinking about changes for the child and the context of the appointment. Is the visit for an ear infection? How will the parents respond if the clinician introduces pharmacotherapy for obesity treatment? Imagine responding to the parents with "Lots of factors help keep us physically and mentally healthy, like good sleep, managing stress, and having friends. What helps keep you healthy? Are there any changes you'd like to make?"

Pashby concluded that to close the gap between the two camps (body positivity and obesity treatment), clinicians must consider how patients feel mentally. How a provider communicates with a patient directly affects how they think and feel; those affect their actions, which influence their behavior, such as physical activity, diet, and sleep. Of course, she said, also follow through with medical treatment, using medications as prescribed, attending medical appointments, and therapy. As one of her patients said, "My ability to do the things that I know are good for my health is tied directly to how I feel mentally."

WHAT TO SAY?

"What are your health goals? Do you have any concerns about your health or how you are feeling that you want to discuss?"

"All bodies are different and unique, and we just want to keep them as healthy as possible. Part of health is your body and your body image, too. How are you feeling about your body?"

"Lots of factors help keep us physically and mentally healthy, like good sleep, managing stress, having friends, staying active and more. What helps keep you healthy? Are there any changes you'd like to make?"

"Are there some ways you think your family can help you feel healthier? Some kids would like more family meals, for example, but that isn't possible for everyone. I am happy to work with all of you to figure it out. It sure can feel hard but you don't have to figure it out alone."

FIGURE 7-4 Sample script for Scenario 3.
SOURCE: Presented by Robyn Pashby, June 26, 2023. Reprinted with permission.

PANEL AND AUDIENCE DISCUSION

Hales led a moderated discussion. The audience asked Essel and Pashby questions about increasing awareness of personal weight bias and stigma among medical faculty, the value of eating less and moving more in obesity treatment, social determinants of health (SDOH), awareness of weight bias and stigma among medical students, and strategies to discuss routine weighing in the clinical setting.

Working with Colleagues to Increase Their Awareness of Weight Bias and Stigma

The first audience question was for Essel, about how he engages and works with colleagues and other faculty who demonstrate weight bias and stigma. After all, the participant commented, students learn from their behavior modeling. Essel responded that the professional dynamic is universal. The team at Children's National Hospital completed chart reviews and found that some language was not up to par. He recalled one example of "buffalo hump" instead of "dorsocervical pad of fat." Or the frequent use of the term "morbid obesity" instead of "severe obesity." The first step, he said, is to think about how to transform the thinking process, posture, and language clinicians use when writing and discussing. The goal is to create a greater awareness of weight bias and stigma among not only students but practicing clinicians. Essel advocated giving providers and medical students the opportunity to hear from families with children who have been affected by the lack of empathy and overt and passive stigma expressed in clinical spaces because it is very effective at raising awareness.

Eat Less and Move More as a Treatment Strategy

The next question from the audience was for Pashby about messaging to eat less and move more in obesity treatment. Does it have a role for patients with obesity? How does it fit into your treatment strategy? Pashby responded that patients have heard this message for decades and internalized it. Why would a clinician reiterate it? Pashby recommended emphasizing activities that the patient loves. That perspective causes a shift from focusing on their body size as unacceptable toward identifying activities that they enjoy.

SDOH and Medical Students

Essel received the next question from the audience about how SDOH influence health care. How does an increased awareness of these affect medical students' perspectives? Essel shared that if faculty teach medical students about SDOH, population health, and public health, then they will have greater awareness and understanding of systems that can lead to increased weight gain and other chronic conditions. However, he continued, that hyper-focusing on SDOH does help students get a better understanding and build empathy, but they can also begin to develop new narratives that indicate obesity is only "acceptable" for those experiencing poverty or who are marginalized. SDOH are critical to understand, but he emphasized the complex models and systems that influence obesity are just as critical. He summarized that obesity risk is more than social risk due to income inequities.

Shifting Away from Routine Weighing in the Clinic: Conversations with Patients

The last question went to Pashby. How can clinicians respond to a patient saying they do not want to be weighed during the office visit? Pashby answered that they should determine if weighing is necessary; it is not at every clinic visit, and they could offer to put a note in the file saying this person prefers not to be weighed. They can also ask about a history of an eating disorder. The likelihood that a person living in a large body has experienced trauma is high. Think about the location of the scale. Is it private or in a high-traffic area? Is weight recorded in the chart or said aloud? Offer to let the patient stand with their back to the scale. Explain why recording their weight is necessary at the visit. Alternatively, ask about a weight on file or any significant weight change since their last visit.

8

Ethics and Trust in Communicating About the Intersection of Body Weight and Health

The third sessions, moderated by Bryn Austin, featured three presentations highlighting ethics and trust when communicating about body weight and health, policies to mitigate poverty in the context of food and health, and cultivating trust in the patient–provider relationship. A panel and audience discussion followed.

WEIGHT-RELATED STIGMA AND HEALTH DISPARITIES

The first presentation was given by Tracy Richmond, director of the Boston Children's Hospital Eating Disorders Outpatient Program and the STEP wellness program for youth with an elevated body mass index (BMI), on weight-related stigma and health disparities. She noted the tension of her roles in the two fields of eating disorders and childhood obesity. To illustrate, she used body acceptance as an example. The field of disordered eating believes that everyone should accept all body sizes and shapes. The field of childhood obesity believes that everyone above a certain number or BMI threshold should lose weight.

Richmond noted that the 2023 American Academy of Pediatrics (AAP) guideline for childhood obesity has received considerable media attention on its recommended interventions, such as weight-loss medications or surgery (Hampl et al., 2023). Less attention has been given to the guidance for patient–provider communication: that clinicians communicate BMI to the patient and their family because it provides rationale for a comprehensive evaluation and treatment of obesity and related comorbidities. However, Richmond cautioned about significant implications.

Richmond shared that public health researchers have documented that many patients with higher weights do not perceive themselves as being overweight. Many clinicians and public health practitioners have blamed this misperception for why public health interventions have not resulted in meaningful outcomes. She detailed the common assumption that if the patient does not recognize weight as problematic, treatment interventions are destined to fail.

Richmond confirmed that some research supports this. One study showed that if patients accurately perceived themselves as overweight, they reported more weight-loss attempts. However, other research has shown that teenagers who were overweight and perceived themselves as so demonstrated fewer healthy behaviors (Hahn et al., 2018) and more internalized weight bias (Puhl et al., 2018); they reported more attempts at weight loss but actually *gained more weight over time* (Haynes et al., 2018).

Richmond also shared results from studies that suggested a protective effect of positive weight perceptions on health. A longitudinal study followed 20,000 people from grades 7–12 into their 40s. Teenagers who were overweight and held positive beliefs about their weight status were less likely to develop disordered eating behaviors (Hazzard et al., 2017; Sonneville et al., 2016a), had lower blood pressure later in life (Unger et al., 2017), fewer depressive symptoms (Thurston et al., 2017), and *gained less weight over time* (Sonneville et al., 2016b).

Richmond admitted that in the beginning of STEP, she and her team documented and notified patients of their weight, spending ample time trying to convince them that it was problematic. The team believed that this was the first step in motivating them to make changes, but in hindsight, this approach was inappropriate and pathologized their weight and body.

Surprisingly, Richmond said, patients pushed back. They expressed very positive feelings about their bodies. The teens said they would be willing to lose some weight so long as it did not change their shape, for example.

This experience led to some ethical questions for Richmond and her team. From the childhood obesity perspective, was it necessary or ethical to increase the child's concern about their weight and make them feel bad about their body? From the eating disorder perspective, was it beneficial for children to feel good about their bodies despite being overweight? Was there something beneficial to them feeling quite good about their bodies?

To explore it further, Richmond's research team surveyed 150 young adults at a university in the southern United States on body satisfaction, and researchers measured their height and weight. Participants also self-identified their body size using a body silhouette scale. Results showed that students accurately reported their BMI based on their self-reported height and weight versus that directly measured by researchers, with no difference in accuracy based on their reported weight perception (i.e., self-reporting themselves to be just about the right weight versus having overweight or obesity). Furthermore, students who scored higher on body satisfaction scales were less likely to self-perceive as having overweight or obesity. Essentially, this study confirmed that individuals are accurate in understanding their weight status but may choose to consider themselves in a more positive light.

Returning to the AAP guidelines to communicate BMI to pediatric patients and their families, Richmond asked why clinicians would (re)tell them, if they are already aware of it. She argued that doing so risks introducing weight stigma and may be more damaging than helpful. Weight stigmatization, she defined, is negative or stereotypical beliefs and social devaluation of people living in large bodies. Weight is cited as the most common reason for youth bullying.

Richmond highlighted research that has shown the negative effects of weight bias and stigma. Psychological health is impacted by weight stigmatization, with greater prevalence of depression and anxiety, lower self-esteem, poor body image, and risk of substance abuse (Hunger and Major, 2015), more binge eating, greater caloric intake, more disordered weight control behaviors, less motivation to exercise, and decreased physical activity (Puhl and Suh, 2015). There are also physical or physiological health consequences of increased cortisol, C-creative protein, blood pressure, and HbA1C and less glycemic control (Tomiyama et al., 2018).

Richmond asserted that communication affects all patients, and weight stigmatization can lead to negative health outcomes in people living in larger bodies. It risks lower quality of care, with reports of contemptuous, patronizing, and disrespectful treatment when interacting with clinicians and health care systems (Alberga et al., 2019; Aldrich and Hackley, 2010; Phelan et al., 2015). Richmond detailed research showing that patients who experience weight stigma had poorer mental health status, increased disordered eating behaviors, and negative physiological health outcomes (Hunger and Major, 2015; Puhl and Suh, 2015; Tomiyama et al., 2018). Doctors are named the second most common source of weight stigma, she said.

Other research, Richmond continued, has shown that providers attribute all health issues to weight when assessing patients living in larger bodies. Physicians make assumptions about behaviors and assume they never exercise or are eating poorly (Alberga et al., 2019; Phelan et al., 2015). She mentioned reports of patients with a sore throat who are lectured about the value of weight loss and physicians spending less time in appointments and building rapport with patients who have overweight or obesity (Aldrich and Hackley, 2010; Phelan et al., 2015). They also receive less screening for cervical, breast, or colorectal cancer and are offered fewer interventions (Aldrich and Hackley, 2010). Offices and hospitals lack right-sized equipment, such as cuffs to measure blood pressure and imaging machines, and have difficulty lifting and moving patients in the operating room (Aldrich and Hackley, 2010; Phelan et al., 2015).

Richmond stated that quality of care is negatively impacted because physicians are not trained to treat patients of various sizes. For example, as a medical student, she was trained to do a PAP smear on a 45-year-old fit White woman. Learning the procedure with someone of a different body size can impact the quality of care of individuals living in larger bodies, potentially contributing to disparities in health care for them.

However, Richmond highlighted a paradigm shift among some clinicians for a weight-inclusive approach as opposed to the traditional weight-normative one (see Figure 8-1), which emphasizes weight loss to achieve health and well-being. Weight is the focal point for interventions, and body size is seen as controllable. Individuals are encouraged to engage in lifestyle changes and behaviors that will lead to weight loss, such as exercise. She detailed that food is considered categorically dichotomous as good or bad, healthy, or unhealthy, should or should not. People are expected to understand their needs based on calories or calorie exchanges.

In contrast, the focal points for intervention in a weight-inclusive approach are health behaviors and social determinants of health (SDOH) rather than an all-or-nothing focus on numbers (Association for Size

Weight Normative vs. Weight Inclusive

	Weight Normative	Weight Inclusive
Weight	• Body size is highly controllable • Individuals should engage in weight control behaviors to achieve a "healthy" weight	• Body size is a morally-neutral, naturally-varying human characteristic • Genetics and social determinants of health >>> individual behaviors
Food	• Good/bad, health/unhealthy, should/shouldn't etc. • Quantity/quality determined by external source (calories, grams, exchanges)	• All food has value and is acceptable • Quantity/quality are determined by responding to physical cues (hunger/fullness, taste, etc.)
Physical activity	• Exercise for weight control	• Be active in fun/enjoyable and functional ways

FIGURE 8-1 Weight-inclusive approach as opposed to the traditional weight-normative approach by clinicians.
SOURCES: Presented by Tracy Richmond, June 26, 2023 (data from http://www.haescommunity.org; https://haescurriculum.com). Reprinted with permission.

Diversity and Health, 2020; Tylka et al., 2014; Weight Inclusive Nutrition and Dietetics, 2023). Body size is morally neutral and recognized as a natural varying human characteristic, so that people of all sizes, ability levels, and health statuses are accepted. Richmond emphasized the focus on genetics and the notion that all food is acceptable and that the quality and quantity of food are determined by taste and hunger and fullness cues.

Richmond encouraged clinicians to consider a weight-inclusive health care practice upheld by three tenets. The first is acknowledging a patient's experience, which can build rapport. Higher-weighted patients likely have had stigmatizing experiences with health care professionals and are hesitant to interact again. Patients likely have tried to lose weight repeatedly, with frustrating results. They may have heightened sensitivity to conversations about weight. The second tenet is for the clinicians to communicate respectfully. They can ask if it is okay to talk about weight and weight-related topics and preferred terms to avoid stigmatization (e.g., "fat" versus "overweight" or "obese"). The last tenet is to focus treatment on behavior, not weight. Richmond emphasized that focusing on weight can contribute to a patient's feelings of shame or frustration and promote extreme or unsustainable weight control strategies.

POVERTY, HEALTH POLICY, AND OBESITY

Martin Wilkinson, professor of politics and international relations at the University of Auckland, was the second presenter and focused on poverty and the uneven distribution of people with obesity among the population.

Wilkinson noted that in high-income countries, such as the United States and New Zealand, people with obesity tend to be low income. Although the distribution of body weight across a community varies by income, the goal would be to mitigate poverty to address inequity. Poverty is a problem in many countries, and several policy options exist to address it. Notably, he said, New Zealand has no farm subsidy policies or food deserts.

Wilkinson distinguished two ways that policy could try to solve the problem of poverty. One would be to give people money through a system that would equate to a welfare system or a labor market where people either have reasonable, secure, and predictable incomes or are ensured jobs that pay reasonably well. He contended that this is a complicated solution.

The second approach is by trying to supervise people's choices, to discourage choices that are bad for them and encourage choices that are good for them. In the context of weight, one line of thinking is to make healthier options less expensive and easier to access. Alternatively, he said, a policy could make unhealthy options more expensive and less accessible through taxes.

One example Wilkinson gave was for a policy to tax sugar, as in the United Kingdom, or dietary fat, as in Hungary. Discouraging unhealthy foods could also be achieved by restricting promotions for junk food (e.g., "buy one, get one free"), restricting unhealthy product displays at stores, or zoning to prevent a high density of fast-food restaurants. These strategies aim to prevent people from purchasing unhealthy products and increase access to healthier products.

Wilkinson hypothesized that if a policy did not work or change behavior, it might increase inequities. For example, the goal of taxing sugar is to raise the price of sugary drinks to dissuade people from purchasing them. If it was ineffective, Wilkinson argued that people would be worse off because they would be paying more and still consuming the same amount of sugar.

Broadening the focus, Wilkinson offered a couple of observations on human behavior. The first is that health is not the predominant value that people equate to a good life. The second is that people often risk their health for another value. For example, Wilkinson highlighted grandparents who often play with their grandchildren, increasing their risk for getting sick. Similarly, professional athletes often set goals that increase their health risk.

In the context of food, Wilkinson noted an avocado shortage in New Zealand. Avocado prices increased to $5–6 USD. Healthy foods are often more expensive and take more time to prepare or cook. If you do not have the money or a kitchen, the alternative is eating unhealthy food that does not need to be prepared ahead of time.

Wilkinson returned to the issue of poverty and inequity. To solve the problem of poverty, he said, policy makers must reform the labor market or introduce a welfare system, and if that is not possible, they can try to change consumer choices and institute policies that influence their purchase decisions. The latter option, he said, could lead to inequitable choices with more expensive, convenient foods and less expensive, inconvenient foods.

COMMUNITY AND PUBLIC TRUST ASPECTS OF COMMUNICATION

The last speaker was Thomas Lee, internist at Brigham and Women's Hospital, chief medical officer of Press Ganey, and professor at the Harvard T.H. Chan School of Public Health. His presentation was about improving the patient–provider relationship by building trust, respect, and hope in the health care system and public system health.

Lee began by asking the audience to consider the elements of trust. What is it, and how do clinicians create it? According to Frances Frei's *The Trust Triangle*, it is built with three components: empathy, authenticity, and logic (Frei and Morriss, 2020). He said that patients must believe the clinician has enduring empathy for them, is authentic and does not forget them after the appointment, and has logic (is able to create a care plan). He emphasized that all three components are required to build trust in the provider or health care system.

For example, Lee shared his work using artificial intelligence and natural language processing to analyze over 2 million patient comments for concepts related to trust, respect, etc. The results showed 35,000 separate insights directly related to trust. He emphasized that patients want to trust their providers and the organizations they engage with.

Lee also noted that the results showed that trust was bidirectional (patients also need to understand that their clinicians trust them). For example, one patient commented that their doctor listened to them, validated their knowledge of their disease, and trusted that they knew their body and how they responded to treatment.

Similarly, Lee's study found that a clinician's failure to convey respect was associated with less trust. Its relevance to health care is that certain features are reliably present when patients have confidence in their provider. Courtesy and respect were especially important to underrepresented minorities in health care, he said. Respect was also found to be bidirectional.

Lee turned the discussion to the concept of hope. Clinicians can create a sense of hope in health care which, in his opinion, is part of quality of life that motivates behavior change. Hope theory has an initial idea of how circumstances will progress and a belief in a positive future. Lee posited that hope lies between what is likely to happen and what could happen. In the context of health, clinicians must have the skill and understand the path between where patients are in their health journey, where they are likely to go, and what might be possible.

Lee posed a question to the audience: how can clinicians and providers reliably offer hope to patients, particularly given no shared identity? To facilitate including hope in the care process, Lee and his colleagues developed a checklist for providers (Mylod and Lee, 2023).

Broadening the topic, Lee recounted the character and lessons of Confucius, who believed that rituals and frequent predictable moments where a person behaves as they should were important. Lee asserted that if a person performs the rituals, they would hone their instincts to anticipate other's needs, gain their trust, give them hope, and motivate them to change their behavior to improve their health. The same is true for clinicians, he said.

PANEL AND AUDIENCE DISCUSSION

After each presentation, Austin led a question-and-answer discussion with the audience. The audience asked Richmond, Wilkinson, and Lee about when it is appropriate to discuss BMI with patients; public health policies and commercial actors; nutrition assistance vouchers in the United States; and trust, respect, and hope in health care for people living in larger bodies.

Situations to Discuss BMI with Patients

The first question was for Richmond: "Could you share the situations in which discussing BMI would be appropriate?" Richmond emphasized that discussing BMI with patients is not all or nothing. Patients have different growth trajectories, so reviewing the patterns is important to look for any changes. Weight in eating disorders is relevant in terms of a pattern change or sudden weight gain. Similarly, a sudden change in weight could reflect a medication change or be an indicator of mental health. In the latter case, Richmond said, clinicians could build rapport and ask if anything has changed in their personal or professional lives.

Focusing on Public Health Policies with Awareness of Upstream Commercial Actors

An audience member commented on Wilkinson's presentation, specifically about patients from historically marginalized groups, and respecting agency and autonomy for their health behaviors, even if they are unhealthy. What advice, they asked, would Wilkinson offer to public health professionals regarding policies and programs that respect people's autonomy and maintain a focus on upstream influences, such as commercial actors or government policies that might limit choices? Wilkinson agreed that respecting agency and autonomy, particularly for those from historically marginalized groups, is paramount. He reiterated that his idea on autonomy was meant for making independent choices, whether good, bad, or in between. Regarding advice on dealing with upstream issues, clinicians must not fall prey to the politician's syllogism: a problem exists, and something must be done that will not make people worse off than before. He urged the audience to seek evidence for people's reactions to a policy. It is easier to justify stopping people from doing things they do not want to do versus what they do.

Nutrition Assistance Vouchers in the United States and Equity

Another question was about Wilkinson's opinion about the restrictions for nutrition assistance vouchers in the United States. Are they equitable? Wilkinson responded that he considered them inequitable. Theoretically, the price is raised so consumers cannot buy a product, which is not equitable. He said people who are receiving assistance are among the worst off in society, and that is not their fault. The question is why not give them more food and beverage options? They could receive money instead of the government offering to pay for healthy foods.

Austin agreed with Wilkinson about the tendency to gravitate toward nutrition-tied assistance as opposed to addressing underlying income inequities.

Trust, Respect, and Hope in Medicine, Clinical Care, and Society

The next question was for Lee: "How do the issues of trust, respect, and hope fit into national efforts to improve diversity, equity, and inclusion in medicine, clinical care, and society?" Lee responded that he thought these concepts were relevant, particularly since the murder of George Floyd; people have worked to understand the difference between treating people equally and the meaning of equity and inclusion. Many organizations have publicly shared their value system for equity, but implementation will take time. Treating people with respect does not cost money, but he asserted that executive leadership must realize the social capital for their entity, whether it be a nursing unit, a health care system, or a company.

Respect in the Medical System: Providing Care for People Living in Larger Bodies

An audience member commented that traditionally, in clinical care, providers thought it was respectful to be truthful and objective when informing patients about the severity and trajectory of their condition. A question for Lee was, what constitutes respect in the context of providing health care for people living in larger bodies? Lee replied that he learned a great deal from the other workshop presentations because of the diversity of speakers and perspectives that he had not been exposed to. Everyone has points of ignorance, he said, and feedback from different people decreases those.

Lee continued that health care delivery has large, institutional gaps in knowledge. For example, a medical school, an elite training program, is reluctant to accept students who have overweight or obesity. The underlying thought is that such a doctor may not help control a patient's risk factors or be a good example. Lee pointed out that this is the equivalent of institutional racism built into the selection of medical students.

The first step he suggested is to acknowledge the issues. Much of the workshop focused on not offending patients. More important, he said, is for clinicians to have effective conversations with people who want to lose weight.

Equity in health care, Lee elaborated, would mean that all patients have a medical exam in the same room or physical space, using the same equipment. He said that equity might be the point that Richmond made about right-sized chairs or blood pressure cuffs.

Lee asked, "What is the goal in health care?" Providers cannot deliver on immortality. The goal is for clinicians to help patients live as long and as well as possible and give them peace of mind that their health is as good as it can be given their circumstances. Lee recommended that clinicians make patients feel that they have listened to their story and concerns, they are respected and trusted, and their clinician is compassionate and trying to meet their needs.

Lee ended by stating that people are heterogeneous, and clinicians must try to meet them where they are to ensure peace of mind. To deliver patient-centered care to individuals, clinicians must understand their biases about different patients regardless of their identity.

9

Improving Communication About Body Weight

The fourth session featured two presentations highlighting the Trust for America's Health (TFAH) and Robert Wood Johnson Foundation (RWJF) and their strategies for improving communication about body weight from a policy and public health perspective. Ihuoma Eneli moderated the session and led a panel and audience discussion afterward.

IMPROVING COMMUNICATION ABOUT BODY WEIGHT FROM A POLICY AND PUBLIC HEALTH PERSPECTIVE: TFAH

J. Nadine Gracia is the president and chief executive officer (CEO) of TFAH, a nonpartisan nonprofit organization that promotes health and ensures that health equity and prevention are foundational in policy making and supported by data and research to improve population health. Gracia gave the first presentation on how TFAH applies communications principles to inform its policy and advocacy efforts for obesity and chronic disease prevention.

Gracia provided an overview of TFAH's advocacy goals to advance and translate evidence into laws and policies that protect and promote health and advance health equity. TFAH "makes the case" to policy makers with evidence-based policy recommendations, data, promising examples and spotlights, stories from the field, and media collaborations to help shape and shift the narrative to advance priorities.

However, Gracia noted, agencies and programs must have sufficient resources to be effective. TFAH also works to secure funding for critical public health investments at the federal level on emerging and long-standing priorities, such as public health infrastructure, emergency preparedness, and obesity prevention. Gracia noted that TFAH informs and engages with policy makers (including Congress and the administration) on key public health priorities, leveraging windows of opportunity and advocating to ensure critical public health issues are addressed.

Gracia emphasized the importance of knowing and understanding the audience and their priorities to help inform policy advocacy strategies. She detailed that TFAH uses several levers for policy engagement in congressional meetings, offering technical assistance on legislation, hosting congressional briefings, and submitting comments in response to requests for information or regulatory actions. The organization informs and communicates with policy makers to understand their perspectives and priorities.

Gracia began by referencing the report *The Impact of Chronic Underfunding on America's Health System* (TFAH, 2023), which outlined that over $4 trillion is spent annually on health, but that does not translate into positive health outcomes (Martin et al., 2023). Only a fraction (about 4–5 percent) is allocated to public health and prevention, and it shows (TFAH, 2022). The United States ranks the lowest in life expectancy compared to other high-income countries (Roser, 2020). Adequate investment in the public health system is critical when advocating for policies promoting healthy people and communities.

Gracia indicated that TFAH's first report on obesity was derived from national priorities. Twenty years ago, the U.S. Surgeon General released a call to action on overweight and obesity to raise awareness among policy makers (HHS, 2001). In response, TFAH launched a report, *F as in Fat*, that highlighted the trends in obesity with data-supported strategies to address it.

Gracia noted that the "F" was intended to describe the failure of policy to address this public health issue and raise awareness. Although the title raised attention, it could also be misinterpreted and inadvertently stigmatize individuals living with obesity. It evolved in 2014 to *The State of Obesity*, recognizing the increased awareness and important progress made and highlighting the data, evidence, programs, and policies to promote optimal health and well-being.

Gracia highlighted that recent reports have included a special feature that elevate critical areas, including racial and ethnic disparities in obesity and advancing health equity; food insecurity and its connection to obesity; and the intersections of the COVID-19 pandemic, social determinants of health (SDOH), and obesity. The 2022 report focuses on food and nutrition insecurity among youth and families, the social and economic conditions that promote food insecurity, and creating policies and systems that promote healthy community conditions (TFAH, 2022).

Gracia shared some lessons that have informed TFAH's approaches and recommendations. Although obesity is a public health issue, multisector action and policy change are critical to progress. She noted key developments from the day's workshop, such as recognizing obesity as a disease, a broader understanding of SDOH, prioritizing health equity by addressing the systemic inequities of structural and systemic discrimination and racism that contribute to health disparities, and further addressing weight-based stigma and discrimination.

Returning to TFAH's communication strategies, Gracia indicated that advocating for obesity prevention policies can be positioned in different ways depending on the audience. It can be a national security issue about military readiness; studies have shown that only one in three military-age people meet the body mass index (BMI) eligibility cutoff determined by the Department of Defense. She continued that it can also be seen through the lens of health equity and nutrition security, and especially for the COVID-19 pandemic, which exacerbated inequities. Neighborhoods with more Black residents had fewer supermarkets and greater food insecurity, but transforming policy and systems is an opportunity to create healthy and resilient communities, she said.

Gracia turned the discussion to TFAH's priorities to adequately fund obesity prevention and public health programs. For example, she pointed to Centers for Disease Control and Prevention (CDC), which receives 31 cents per person for evidence-based obesity prevention programs, such as its effective State Physical Activity and Nutrition program (CDC, 2023; grants.gov, 2018). Gracia explained that the consequence is that funding is only sufficient for 16 states; the other 34 states and the U.S. territories are excluded. CDC program funding has been stagnant and not kept pace with the magnitude of obesity (CDC, 2023).

Gracia highlighted that TFAH reports demonstrate the data for overweight and obesity at the population level and inform policy makers that it is a complex, multifaceted issue in need of addressing. Broader community conditions, such as issues of poverty, health insurance coverage, participation in Supplemental Nutrition Assistance Program (SNAP), and examining the proportion of the eligible population that is participating, provide a more comprehensive picture of structural drivers of obesity for policy makers.

Gracia ended by revisiting the notion of seizing the moment to inform the administration's priorities. The school meal programs, for example, stem from the 1946 National School Lunch Act to the 2010 Healthy and Hunger-Free Kids Act and aim to improve school nutrition standards and increase access to healthy school meals to reduce obesity, especially for children living in households with low incomes. Gracia urged participants to leverage the opportunity and momentum created by the Biden–Harris administration's National Strategy on Hunger, Nutrition, and Health (White House, 2022) to advocate and educate policy makers on obesity prevention and treatment, emphasizing SDOH.

A NEW NARRATIVE ON CHILDHOOD OBESITY

Jennie Day-Burget was the second speaker and presented on the progression of narratives about obesity at RWJF, where she is the senior communications officer. She shared that RWJF is building a national culture of health, rooted in equity, to provide all people with opportunity for health and well-being no matter who they are, where they live, or how much money they have.

Day-Burget opened by indicating that RWJF is shifting away from individual responsibility and blame for obesity and working to change policies and the environment. Recently, she said, it has learned about the inadvertent impact of words and acknowledges the prevailing narratives on childhood obesity that have unintentionally contributed to and exacerbated anti-fat bias in children. Feelings of shame, sadness, and embarrassment have been found to be connected to terms such as "fat" and "weight problem" among children. Although "epidemic" and "disease" are found in the media and doctor's offices, raising the profile of the health impacts of obesity, the same language has led to toxic connections between bodies with obesity and diseases (Kyle and Puhl, 2014; Puhl et al., 2017).

In the past, Day-Burget said that TFAH and RWJF cobranded the report, *F as in Fat*. The goal of the title was to use shock language to garner media attention to spark a conversation about policy and system changes to address obesity prevention. She explained that by doing so and focusing on the deep and persistent disparities of childhood obesity rates, the report called attention to a public health challenge faced by many communities. However, it did not describe the positive attributes of those same communities; although it received plenty of media coverage, it caused harm.

Day-Burget outlined the steps that RWJF has taken to improve the narrative about obesity. The foundation has launched an annual report, the *State of Childhood Obesity*, telling families' stories and sharing personal narratives to animate the data. She continued that RWJF no longer focuses on obesity-rate data and instead promotes the perspectives of the community thought leaders and emphasizes systems-level solutions that could improve the built environment for better health. She added that RWJF has also shifted to using people-first language, not blaming individuals, and refocusing on systems change.

Day-Burget turned to discuss media and childhood obesity. To better understand the impact of the COVID-19 pandemic on such narratives, RWJF analyzed popular media outlets (e.g., Twitter) and coverage on obesity, stigma, and bias. The goal was to understand how obesity and weight stigma were depicted in the media through language and the primary messengers. Although the findings showed a regression to individual responsibility and blame, other results showed progress. The media began shifting to positive language, emphasizing a shift in cultural norms. Unfortunately, she said, findings also showed that social media used traditional language about obesity. With high engagement rates, social media promotes purposefully offensive, negative discussions about weight.

Day-Burget illustrated the self-reflection at RWJF by sharing its study on the language of structural racism and health over 14 months to understand how to engage audiences in discussion about structural racism and health and possibly act. The results generated a formula of three parts to engage persuadable audiences to communicate about obesity and weight, particularly with structural racism as the underlying system: a shared, values-based ideal statement, positive vision and problem statement, and call to action and unity statement. RWJF applied this formula to a script for social media influencers on summer hunger that begins with a shared value statement:

> We all want to live in a country where our children and grandchildren go to sleep each night with full bellies, a country where kids have easy access to healthy foods no matter how much money their families make, what they look like or where they live (shared value statement). But this is not everyone's reality. That is because there are barriers built in front of some of us that create unequal opportunity, freedom, and prosperity. For millions of children, unequal opportunity will be felt acutely this summer, the time of year they most often go hungry because kids are out of school and lose access to consistent, healthy school meals. This comes at a time when many of their families are also struggling with the rising costs of food (problem statement). If your PTA or school community has not yet shared how to access summer meals for kids, please encourage them to do so and share this link with them. Since people created the laws and social practices that shape these opportunities, we can reinvent them. We can work together so that everyone's children and grandchildren have the best possible future, and everyone can reach their best health and well-being (call to action and unity statement). (Robert Wood Johson Foundation)

Day-Burget noted that the same communications principles can help to depict structural racism in health through a static image (see Figure 9-1).

Day-Burget ended by reiterating RWJF's commitment to examine and continuously improve its approach to create narratives for better communication about childhood obesity that promotes unity and refrains from perpetuating stigma and harm.

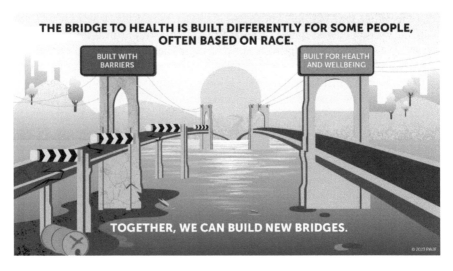

FIGURE 9-1 Image depicting structural racism in health.
SOURCES: Presented by Jennie-Day-Burget, June 26, 2023; RWJF, 2023. Reprinted with permission.

PANEL AND AUDIENCE DISCUSION

Eneli thanked the presenters for sharing practical strategies and complimented their organizations and leadership for their bravery in recognizing missteps with good intentions. Eneli then led a moderated discussion with questions from the audience for Gracia and Day-Burget about lessons learned for effective and trustworthy communication with communities.

Lessons Learned: Effective Communication Factors

Eneli began with a question for Gracia and Day-Burget. Thinking about TFAH and RWJF's policies and initiatives, which have had the most success in terms of the communication strategies? Are there tips that the audience could apply in their work?

Day-Burget responded first and said that shifting from personal responsibility to policy systems and the environment for obesity prevention refocused the RWJF narrative that consumers can only choose options that they have. It acknowledges individual responsibility and the system and has been well received. One surprise, she said, was the backslide observed in their research during the pandemic, emphasizing that progress is fragile.

Gracia shared that TFAH found an effective communications strategy that goes beyond simply data points to describe barriers and why they may exist. It created new dialogues using person-first language and provided greater context that humanizes the discussion. During the pandemic, messages on food insecurity were effective because so many families and communities were at risk and a broader understanding existed of the connection between access to nutritious foods and the risk for obesity. Gracia continued that the narrative shifted to ensure that communities and families have access to resources and opportunities to be healthy and highlighted success stories. Sharing on-the-ground experience humanizes the data points and has been critically important in understanding the need for equitable access to affordable, healthy food and economic opportunities, she said.

Eneli followed up with a question for Day-Burget and RWJF. Did the study identify societal factors that led to backsliding? Day-Burget replied that it did not but that research at RWJF tested messages on SNAP participants, focusing on the concept that a hand up is not a handout. A campaign with storytelling, media partnerships, and work with Mathematica promoted evidence-based research about the impact of potential changes to SNAP on families was powerful and effective.

Lessons Learned: Effectively Using Data in Messaging

An audience member commented that they had been advocating for expanding nutrition services through Medicaid in DC and struggled with data access. Do TFAH or RWJF have state-by-state policies on Medicaid?

Gracia highlighted one of TFAH's policy recommendations is expanding access to health care coverage, including Medicaid expansion in remaining states. Gracia responded that these data need to be disaggregated to improve completeness for public health and health care. It is paramount to have access to robust data to make informed decisions and ensure resources are equitably allocated to communities. Day-Burget added that RWJF is working to expand Medicaid on the state level. It is moving away from data disparities and narratives and toward contextualizing data. RWJF's research showed that leading with these narratives about families and children can be harmful.

Lessons Learned: Trust and Communication

A final question from the audience was about trust and communication: "How do TFAH and RWJF handle miscommunication in social media?"

Day-Burget began by stating that RWJF is monitoring social media, trying to figure out what to do about misinformation and disinformation, although she emphasized the lack of an easy solution. It is also undertaking organizational reflection about past messaging campaigns that unintentionally harmed children and their families.

Gracia added that TFAH is actively engaged in work on countering misinformation, particularly during the COVID-19 pandemic. In 2020, TFAH launched the Public Health Communications Collaborative with the de Beaumont Foundation and CDC Foundation, offering messaging guidance and resources to state and local health departments and health officials. Its website has a misinformation tracker that guides users on how or whether to respond.

Misinformation and disinformation are ongoing issues in public health. Gracia emphasized the importance of earning trust for effective communication, building authentic and meaningful partnerships with trusted messengers from local communities, and listening to and learning about individual and community concerns so that messages are pertinent, tailored, and nonjudgmental.

10

Promoting Change in Culture and Perception About Body Weight

The fifth and final session, moderated by Nico Pronk, included two presentations on strategies to promote culture change and perceptions about body weight. A moderated discussion and question-and-answer period with participants followed.

A SOCIOECOLOGICAL APPROACH TO ADDRESSING STRUCTURAL RACISM AND WEIGHT DISCRIMINATION

The first presentation was on the intersection of structural racism and weight discrimination using a sociocultural or socioecological approach. Natalie Slopen, an assistant professor in the Department of Social and Behavioral Sciences at the Harvard T.H. Chan School of Public Health and affiliated faculty member at the Center on the Developing Child at Harvard University, introduced the socioecological model (SEM) (Bronfenbrenner, 1979) to guide the presentation and the systems of oppression for structural racism and obesity stigma.

Slopen referenced SEM, which nests layers of systems for the developing individual across a lifetime. She described additional layers for children, who may be nested in a family unit, school setting, community, and state, which may have policies that impact one another.

Slopen asserted that many interconnected systems of structural racism exist in medicine and health care, education, banking, and housing and neighborhoods. She explained that the systems have downstream implications and consequences for if and how people interact with each other, which impacts their health and development across a lifetime. SEM also identifies areas and places to address inequities through interventions, she said.

Slopen underscored that "structural racism shapes the environment in which people grow up, learn, work, and play, affecting access to healthy foods, a safe environment, and physical activity." She continued that it has created and perpetuated inequitable social environments, shaped social determinants of health (SDOH), and led to the discriminatory treatment of minoritized individuals, resulting in differences in body size and long-term health:

> The totality of ways in which societies foster racial discrimination through mutually reinforcing systems [...]. These patterns and practices in turn reinforce discriminatory beliefs, values, and distribution of resources. (Bailey et al., 2017)

Slopen explained that structural racism contributes to racial and ethnic disparities in health; marginalized communities have a higher prevalence of obesity because of their limited access to affordable nutritious food in their neighborhoods, more marketing of unhealthy food, limited access to safe places for physical activity, etc.

Slopen asserted that some researchers believe socioeconomic status can wholly explain neighborhood patterns, although racism is central. To illustrate, she presented data on U.S. children residing in poverty, stratified by levels in Dolores Acevedo-Garcia's *Child Opportunity Index*, a metric developed to characterize contextual advantages and disadvantages for children's health that ranks neighborhoods based on 29 dimensions of opportunity, such as the number and quality of schools, early education centers, graduation rates, home ownership, green space, healthy food outlets, and walkability.

Slopen highlighted that the differences in the environment cannot be explained by income. When she filtered the data for children living below the poverty line, she found striking disparities: 66 percent of poor Black children and 50 percent of poor Hispanic Latino children live in neighborhoods with very low opportunity compared to 20 percent of White children (Acevedo-Garcia et al., 2020).

Slopen shifted to focus on discriminatory treatment that minoritized individuals endure due to their multiple social identities. She explained that the intersection of structural racism and obesity stigma overlap and serve as independent sources of discrimination and disadvantage or preference and advantage for subgroups. People stigmatized for their overlapping social identities face compounded effects on their health and well-being.

Slopen shared four priorities to address the stark disparities in environment and health outcomes. First, she emphasized the importance of comprehensive approaches to address the root causes of structural racism and obesity stigma. The second priority is to design equitable social and structural environments for all communities. The third is to develop strategies that foster awareness, empathy, and understanding to challenge weight-related bias and stigma. The fourth is to create strategies that inspire political will and commitment for a more equitable future.

A LIVED-EXPERIENCE PERSPECTIVE ON THE CULTURE AND PERCEPTION ABOUT BODY WEIGHT

Brian Castrucci, president and chief executive officer (CEO) of the de Beaumont Foundation and public health advocate with lived experience, was the final presenter. He shared his story as a person who has lived his entire life with obesity, from childhood to adulthood.

He gained and lost weight throughout his life and experienced ridicule and stigma from providers. He recalled losing 50 pounds as a 13-year-old. At his next doctor's visit, his pediatrician did not encourage him but rather said that he was still fat and needed to lose more weight. Castrucci remembers that experience vividly from 36 years ago, and it shaped his future relationship with health care providers; he did not go to the doctor as often as he should, fearing he would be stigmatized and ridiculed.

Castrucci described how weight stigma persists in U.S. culture. He suffered from a heart attack in adulthood and worked hard to lose 70 pounds. When he visited with his endocrinologist, his doctor commented that he was still fat and needed to lose more weight.

According to Castrucci, the pervasive and persistent acceptance of weight stigma is palpable. To illustrate his point, Castrucci searched the Internet for the term "conversion therapy" (which aims to convert children who identify as LGBTQ to be heteronormative). His search yielded results of several websites condemning it and offering support. Castrucci then searched the Internet for the term "fat camp." The first result advertised "the best fat camp for families…" Castrucci stressed the blatant difference in how society and culture view overweight and obesity in children versus other forms of therapy that try to change children.

Castrucci highlighted that this is partly due to the medicalization of obesity that shifted the blame to individuals, like the medicalization of drug use. Demedicalizing language, actions, and policies would require acknowledging SDOH as critical in determining housing, salary, and availability of healthy foods and directly impacting nutrition and possibly weight, he said.

Castrucci said that he thinks about how to feed his children healthy foods. As a CEO of a private philanthropy, he admitted that he has the privilege to live near his workplace in an expensive housing market, whereas some of his staff live 1 hour away, meaning they have 1 hour less to cook dinner, clean up, and get ready for the next day. Castrucci emphasized that the intersectionality of housing costs, salary, and housing availability impacts how parents feed their children, their nutrition, weight, and health.

Castrucci called out an earlier comment that misinformation in medicine only happened during the COVID-19 pandemic. Castrucci pointed to social media advertisements that prey on fears (e.g., "Overnight ways to lose weight," keto or low-carbohydrate diets). Castrucci noted that conflicting information from influencers, who are not experts, has proliferated with social media, but misinformation has always been an issue. He said that to have obesity is a deep fear, with a societal resistance to change.

Castrucci then posed a paradox to demonstrate that health information is not valued or regulated in the United States. He gave the example that if a layperson were to open a primary care clinic, they would go to jail for impersonating a physician. However, it is legal for them to give nutrition advice without any training in nutrition. Castrucci closed by asking the audience:

> How do we shape a society that allows people to be healthy at every weight, prioritizes health, and gives people the information they need to make healthy choices? It is about health, and there is health at every weight.

PANEL AND AUDIENCE DISCUSSION

Pronk led the audience and panel in a moderated discussion. Questions from the audience focused on SEM when planning interventions, trust and shared values concerning people living with obesity, and reasons for low attendance at healthy eating classes.

Using SEM in Interventions

The first question was for Slopen. When applying SEM to understand and address health disparities, how can it be incorporated into interventions?

Slopen replied that SEM applies across the life span. She said to consider how individuals' lives connect with one another across generations, within families, and their communities when planning an intervention. The social environments and structures that impact individuals are distinct and unique, she continued, and neighborhoods may be more influential than the work environment. Slopen said that the challenge is determining the best leverage point.

Building a Language That Prioritizes Chronic Disease

The next question was for Castrucci. Health communication is core to public health. How has it worked in campaigns for chronic health concerns, such as obesity? Castrucci answered that it is necessary to build a language. He pointed to the presentation from Day-Burget about RWJF's work to build a language that prioritizes chronic disease rather than blaming the individual. Castrucci recalled his son coming home after school asking him about his diet. He responded that it was okay and questioned why his son was asking. His son had learned in class that all people with type 2 diabetes have bad diets. Castrucci said that even though this is scientifically inaccurate, that narrative is being built in schools, and elsewhere, with our youngest children. This belief will be difficult to deprogram, he said.

Castrucci continued by talking about how through criminalization and medicalization, U.S. culture has shifted responsibility to the individual and away from society. The diet industry or the vitamin and supplement industry are the biggest purveyors of misinformation, he said. As an example, ivermectin and hydroxychloroquine were advertised to treat COVID-19, which is factually incorrect yet appeared on the front page of a newspaper. Castrucci continued with the example of diet misinformation, and how Dexatrim and other weight-loss drugs are treated with equal veracity, when they should not be. Castrucci also pointed to how the diabetes drug, Ozempic, has been difficult for him to get as a diabetic because it is also being prescribed off label for weight loss and is constantly in the news. U.S. culture prioritizes thin bodies as the normative ideal and when obesity is medicalized, people are showing their disease all day, Castrucci said.

Trust, Shared Values, and People Living in Larger Bodies

Pronk followed up with a comment and question to Castrucci and Slopen. The idea of shared values from the Robert Wood Johnson Foundation (RWJF) seems to make sense when thinking about people as well as societal organizations and government. In the context of SEM, how can shared values be identified? How can clinicians create an authentic and trustworthy dialogue to uncover shared values across different levels of SEM?

Slopen responded that she believes shared values exist and can be identified through more dialogue and cross-sector collaborations. Some organizations are working in silos, and strategic connections could reveal their shared values, she said.

Castrucci agreed that the shared values model works well but pointed out that larger bodies are not accepted in U.S. culture; the shared value is that they should be eradicated. He noted the example of Jack Black, who became a leading man in movies after he lost weight. Castrucci asserted that leading men cannot be overweight. He added two more examples of entertainers who became more desirable after they lost weight: the actor Brendan Fraser and the singer Adele. Castrucci added that it is not a shared value among grandparents for their grandchildren's bodies to be any size or a larger size. Castrucci urged clinicians, scientists, and others to be thoughtful and honest when talking about shared values. It is still acceptable to openly mock people living in larger bodies, he said.

Reasons for Low Attendance at Healthy Eating Classes

An audience member introduced herself as a registered dietitian and long-time educator and shared that she has trouble getting people to attend her healthy eating classes that focus on habits and do not discuss diets, weight, etc. She asked Slopen and Castrucci for their reactions.

Castrucci responded that when he had his heart attack, he was prescribed cardiac rehabilitation, which was inconvenient and time intensive. He said that no one asked how he would fit 108 hours (three times a week for 12 weeks) into his work schedule or travel to and from the facility. He was congratulated by medical professionals who told him that most patients who have a heart attack do not go to cardiac rehabilitation. Castrucci admitted that he could do so because of his privilege as an economically stable White man, not because of diet or exercise.

Castrucci wagered that virtual participants in this workshop were likely working on three tasks while listening into his presentation. He conceded that it is hard to find time for health and that people learn and engage more on social media, such as TikTok. Castrucci highlighted that stress is the culprit of poor health, with demands from children, partners, and spouses. He said that diabetes, chronic disease, and obesity happen over a long period, and people have other immediate priorities to address, such as rent, getting kids to a field trip, or figuring out a partner or spouse's calendar. Castrucci underscored that health care professionals must be more thoughtful about how to make education and trainings more accessible and easier to attend. He summarized by quoting author Michael Pollan: "make the healthy choice the easy choice."

Slopen said that people may not feel comfortable in a healthy eating class. She was reminded of the personal stories from the workshop of people who have had negative experiences in health care and are hesitant to attend such events, fearful they will be singled out or embarrassed. Slopen urged health professionals to think about how they can design programs that create trust, so people feel comfortable about attending.

Castrucci pointed out that characters in movies drive the narrative with obesity. Castrucci explained the societal context using the example of the Little Mermaid: Ariel is an attractive, young, and innocent mermaid, and Ursula is the heavy, ugly sea witch with a low voice. Until racism, sexism, or ableism are broken down, the United States will not make progress, he said.

CLOSING REMARKS

Pronk delivered the final remarks. He recalled that the workshop began with presentations that outlined the problems with using body mass index (BMI) as a clinical parameter. The diagnostic term "obesity" must be redefined and reconceptualized using the criteria established by the American Medical Association: (1) signs or symptoms, (2) harm or morbidity, and (3) dysregulation of body functions. Standardized criteria coupled with a clinical and functional staging system could specify the severity and related complications for a more precise diagnosis, leading to more targeted and efficient strategies to prevent and treat it. Pronk emphasized that scientific evidence must be translated for medically actionable clinical treatment in the International Classification of Diseases, Tenth Revision coding system that directs treatment and reimbursement for clinicians.

Pronk also highlighted the George Washington University curriculum for medical students or learners to recognize their bias and stigma. He reminded the audience of the results from an anonymous self-assessment that jarred medical students who attended the Public Health Summit on Obesity. Pronk highlighted that students experienced a range of reactions, such as denial and overt bias, which aligns with the goal of the summit to grow awareness of weight bias in the clinical field and refocus health care treatment on improving health through 10 steps.

Pronk reiterated that weight bias and stigma extend beyond the clinical setting and are pervasive in U.S. culture, marginalizing people living in large bodies. It is socially acceptable in the United States to view bodies with overweight or obesity as problematic. He was reminded of the example of online advertisements for summer "fat camps" for children and families. It is paradoxical, Pronk stated, that other programs, such as conversion therapy, are unacceptable in U.S. culture.

Broadening the scope, Pronk discussed the paradigm shift in the clinical field. He explained that the goal of the traditional weight-normative approach emphasizes weight and weight loss to achieve health. Pronk shared the modernized weight-inclusive approach that aims to improve a person's health and well-being through various other strategies.

According to Pronk, the evidence was clear that clinicians must communicate more compassionately and effectively. He recalled the presentations that pointed to the language and words clinicians use to discuss obesity, overweight, and health that are linked to behavior and health outcomes. Pronk underlined people-first language as a starting point. Although clinicians have a technical understanding of obesity, he said, they may not know how to talk to their patients. This is partly due to the prevailing narrative that body size is a personal responsibility and obesity results from a lack of restraint—the shift in perspective centers on the role of systems and the environment. Pronk recalled the RWJF evidence-based communication strategy that adjusts the narrative on obesity and health to focus on shared values using three steps to create messages and images.

Pronk noted that research shows that ethics and trust are paramount in health and that patients want to trust their providers. For such a relationship, he reiterated that three elements must be present: authenticity, empathy, and logic. Pronk pointed to the research showing a bidirectional relationship with trust, meaning the more courteous and respectful a provider is to their patient and trusts their patient's perspective and opinion, the more the patient trusts them.

Pronk stated that policy and political will must be required to change the perceptions of overweight and obesity in U.S. society and culture. He reminded participants that the nation has one of the lowest life expectancy rates of high-income countries worldwide because public health programs are underfunded. Pronk shared the desperate need to educate and advocate to decision makers on funding public health adequately and emphasized Trust for America's Health's effective communication strategy through storytelling with people and data to "make the case" for it.

Policy work is complicated, Pronk said, and some policies that aim to improve equity could unintentionally lead to inequitable circumstances, such as the SNAP-related policy that aims to dissuade the purchase of sugar-sweetened beverages by increasing the price. However, if consumers continue to buy them at a higher price point, they will spend more money and not purchase healthier beverages, which would be inequitable.

Pronk underscored the broader context of structural racism and obesity stigma as interconnected systems of oppression that perpetuate harm. He pointed to SEM as a means to identify critical points and issues for study and intervention. Pronk concluded by outlining the priorities to address structural racism and obesity stigma through a comprehensive approach using strategies to foster awareness, empathy, and understanding and a political will that addresses the root causes to create a more equitable future for all.

References

Acevedo-Garcia, D., C. Noelke, N. McArdle, N. Sofer, E. F. Hardy, M. Weiner, M. Baek, N. Huntington, R. Huber, and J. Reece. 2020. Racial and ethnic inequities in children's neighborhoods: Evidence from the new Child Opportunity Index 2.0. *Health Affairs (Millwood)* 39(10):1693–1701.

AHRQ (Agency for Healthcare Research and Quality). 2021. *Strength, Weakness, Opportunities, and Threats Analysis*. https://digital.ahrq.gov/health-it-tools-and-resources/evaluation-resources/workflow-assessment-health-it-toolkit/all-workflow-tools/swot-analysis (accessed October 20, 2023).

Alberga, A. S., B. J. Pickering, K. Alix Hayden, G. D. C. Ball, A. Edwards, S. Jelinski, S. Nutter, S. Oddie, A. M. Sharma, and S. Russell-Mayhew. 2016. Weight bias reduction in health professionals: A systematic review. *Clinical Obesity* 6(3):175–188.

Alberga, A. S., I. Y. Edache, M. Forhan, and S. Russell-Mayhew. 2019. Weight bias and health care utilization: A scoping review. *Primary Health Care Research and Development* 20(e116):1–14.

Aldrich, T., and B. Hackley. 2010. The impact of obesity on gynecologic cancer screening: An integrative literature review. *Journal of Midwifery & Women's Health* 55(4):344–356.

Apovian, C. M., L. J. Aronne, D. H. Bessesen, M. E. McDonnell, M. H. Murad, U. Pagotto, D. H. Ryan, and C. D. Still. 2015. Pharmacological management of obesity: An Endocrine Society Clinical Practice Guideline. *The Journal of Clinical Endocrinology and Metabolism* 100(2):342–362.

Association for Size Diversity and Health. 2020. *About Health at Every Size*. https://asdah.org/health-at-every-size-haes-approach (accessed September 15, 2023).

Austin, S. B., and T. K. Richmond. 2022. It's time to retire BMI as a clinical metric. *Medpage Today*. https://www.medpagetoday.com/opinion/second-opinions/101296 (accessed October 20, 2023).

Baig, K., S. B. Dusetzina, D. D. Kim, and A. A. Leech. 2023. Medicare Part D coverage of antiobesity medication—challenges and uncertainty ahead. *New England Journal of Medicine* 388(11):961–963.

Bailey, Z. D., N. Krieger, M. Agénor, J. Graves, N. Linos, and M. T. Bassett. 2017. Structural racism and health inequities in the USA: Evidence and interventions. *Lancet* 389:1453–1463.

Blayney, D. W. 2008. Strengths, weaknesses, opportunities, and threats. *Journal of Oncology Practice* 4(2):53.

Blüher, M. 2020. Metabolically healthy obesity. *Endocrine Reviews* 41(3):bnaa004.

Bosy-Westphal, A., and M. J. Müller. 2021. Diagnosis of obesity based on body composition–associated health risks—Time for a change in paradigm. *Obesity Reviews*. 22(S2):e13190.

Braveman, P., E. Arkin, T. Orleans, D. Proctor, and A. Plough. 2017. *What is health equity? And what difference does a definition make?* Princeton, NJ: Robert Wood Johnson Foundation.

Bronfenbrenner, U. 1979. *The ecology of human development: Experiments by nature and design*. Cambridge, MA: Harvard University Press.

Brown, A., and S. W. Flint. 2021. Preferences and emotional response to weight-related terminology used by healthcare professionals to describe body weight in people living with overweight and obesity. *Clinical Obesity* 11(5):e12470.

Caban, A. J., D. J. Lee, L. E. Fleming, O. Gómez-Marín, W. LeBlanc, and T. Pitman. 2005. Obesity in U.S. workers: The National Health Interview Survey, 1986 to 2002. *American Journal of Public Health* 95(9):1614–1622.

CDC (Centers for Disease Control and Prevention). 2020. *BRFSS Prevalence and Trends Data*. https://nccd.cdc.gov/BRFSSPrevalence/rdPage.aspx?rdReport=DPH_BRFSS.ExploreByTopic&irbLocationType=StatesAndMMSA&islClass=CLASS14&islTopic=TOPIC09&islYear=2020&rdRnd=62773 (accessed October 20, 2023).

CDC. 2022. *Prevalence of Diagnosed Diabetes*. https://www.cdc.gov/diabetes/data/statistics-report/diagnosed-diabetes.html (accessed October 20, 2023).

CDC, Division of Nutrition, Physical Activity, and Obesity. 2023. *State Physical Activity and Nutrition (SPAN) Program*. https://www.cdc.gov/nccdphp/dnpao/state-local-programs/span-1807/ (accessed October 20, 2023).

Cherian, S., G. D. Lopaschuk, and E. Carvalho. 2012. Cellular cross-talk between epicardial adipose tissue and myocardium in relation to the pathogenesis of cardiovascular disease. *American Journal of Physiology—Endocrinology and Metabolism* 303(8):E937–49.

Clark, S., A. Rene, W. M. Theurer, and M. Marshall. 2002. Association of body mass index and health status in firefighters. *Journal of Occupational and Environmental Medicine* 44(10):940–946.

CMS (Centers for Medicare & Medicaid Services). 2011. *National Coverage Determination: Intensive Behavioral Therapy for Obesity*. https://www.cms.gov/medicare-coverage-database/view/ncd.aspx?NCDId=353 (accessed October 20, 2023).

Deloitte Access Economics, Dove, and STRIPED (Strategic Training Initiative for the Prevention of Eating Disorders: A Public Health Incubator). 2022. *The Real Cost of Beauty Ideals*. https://www.hsph.harvard.edu/striped/wp-content/uploads/sites/1267/2022/10/Real-Cost-of-Beauty-Report-10-4-22.pdf (accessed October 20, 2023).

Eisenberg, D., S. A. Shikora, E. Aarts, A. Aminian, L. Angrisani, R. V. Cohen, M. De Luca, S. L. Faria, K. P. S. Goodpaster, A. Haddad, J. M. Himpens, L. Kow, M. Kurian, K. Loi, K. Mahawar, A. Nimeri, M. O'Kane, P. K. Papasavas, J. Ponce, J. S. A. Pratt, A. M. Rogers, K. E. Steele, M. Suter, and S. N. Kothari. 2022. American Society for Metabolic and Bariatric Surgery (ASMBS) and International Federation for the Surgery of Obesity and Metabolic Disorders (IFSO): Indications for Metabolic and Bariatric Surgery. *Surgery for Obesity and Related Disease* 18(12):1345–1356. https://doi.org/10.1016/j.soard.2022.08.013.

Eknoyan, G. 2008. Adolphe Quetelet (1796–1874) —The average man and indices of obesity. *Nephrology Dialysis Transplantation* 23(1):47–51.

Flegal, K. M., C. L. Ogden, J. A. Yanovski, D. S. Freedman, J. A. Shepherd, B. I. Graubard, and L. G. Borrud. 2010. High adiposity and high body mass index–for-age in U.S. children and adolescents overall and by race-ethnic group, *The American Journal of Clinical Nutrition* 91(4):1020–1026.

Frei, F. X., and A. Morriss. 2020. Begin with trust. *Harvard Business Review*, May–June 2020. https://hbr.org/2020/05/begin-with-trust (accessed August 10, 2023).

Garvey, W. T., A. J. Garber, J. I. Mechanick, G. A. Bray, S. Dagogo-Jack, D. Einhorn, G. Grunberger, Y. Handelsman, C. H. Hennekens, D. L. Hurley, J. McGill, P. Palumbo, G. Umpierrez, and the AACE Obesity Scientific Committee. 2014. American Association of Clinical Endocrinologists and American College of Endocrinology position statement on the 2014 advanced framework for a new diagnosis of obesity as a chronic disease. *Endocrine Practice* 20(9):977–989.

Garvey, W. T., J. I. Mechanick, E. M. Brett, A. J. Garber, D. L. Hurley, A. M. Jastreboff, K. Nadolsky, R. Pessah-Pollack, R. Plodkowski, and Reviewers of the AACE/ACE Obesity Clinical Practice Guidelines. 2016. American Association of Clinical Endocrinologists and American College of Endocrinology comprehensive clinical practice guidelines for medical care of patients with obesity. *Endocrine Practice* 22(Suppl 3):1–203.

Garvey, W. T., and J. I. Mechanick. 2020. Proposal for a scientifically-correct and medically-actionable disease classification system (ICD) for obesity. *Obesity* 28(3):484–492.

Georgetown University Center on Education and the Workforce. 2018. *Shifts in Employment Share for All Industries*. https://cew.georgetown.edu/cew-reports/manufacturingstates/ (accessed October 20, 2023).

Grants.gov. 2018. *CDC-RFA-DP18-1807: State Physical Activity and Nutrition Program: Department of Health and Human Services: Centers for Disease Control—NCCDPHP*. https://www.grants.gov/web/grants/view-opportunity.html?oppId=299540 (accessed October 20, 2023).

Green, B. L., P. A. Saunders, E. Power, P. Dass-Brailsford, K. B. Schelbert, E. Giller, L. Wissow, A. Hurtado-de-Mendoza, and M. Mete. 2015. Trauma-informed medical care: A CME communication training for primary care providers. *Family Medicine* 47(1):7–14.

Gu, J. K., L. E. Charles, K. M. Bang, C. C. Ma, M. E. Andrew, J. M. Violanti, and C. M. Burchfiel. 2014. Prevalence of obesity by occupation among U.S. workers: The National Health Interview Survey 2004–2011. *Journal of Occupational and Environmental Medicine* 56(5):516–528.

Guo, F., D. R. Moellering, and W. T. Garvey. 2014. The progression of cardiometabolic disease: Validation of a new cardiometabolic disease staging system applicable to obesity. *Obesity* 22(1):110–118.

Hadjiyannakis, S., A. Buchholz, J.-P. Chanoine, M. M. Jetha, L. Gaboury, J. Hamilton, C. Birken, K. M. Morrison, L. Legault, T. Bridger, S. R. Cook, J. Lyons, A. M. Sharma, and G. D. C. Ball. 2016. The Edmonton Obesity Staging System for Pediatrics: A proposed clinical staging system for paediatric obesity. *Paediatrics & Child Health* 21(1):21–26.

Hadjiyannakis, S., Q. Ibrahim, J. Li, G. D. C. Ball, A. Buchholz, J. K. Hamilton, I. Zenlea, J. Ho, L. Legault, A-M. Laberge, L. Thabane, M. Tremblay, and K. M. Morrison. 2019. Obesity class versus the Edmonton Obesity Staging System for Pediatrics to define health risk in childhood obesity: Results from the CANPWR cross-sectional study. *The Lancet Child and Adolescent Health* 3(6):398–407.

Hahn, S. L., K. A. Borton, and K. R. Sonneville. 2018. Cross-sectional associations between weight-related health behaviors and weight misperception among U.S. adolescents with overweight/obesity. *BMC Public Health* 18(1):1–8.

Hales, C. M., C. D. Fryar, M. D. Carroll, D. S. Freedman, and C. L. Ogden. 2018. Trends in obesity and severe obesity prevalence in U.S. youth and adults by sex and age, 2007–2008 to 2015–2016. *Journal of the American Medical Association* 319(16):1723–1725.

Hamman, R. F., R. R. Wing, S. L. Edelstein, J. M. Lachin, G. A. Bray, L. Delahanty, M. Hoskin, A. M. Kriska, E. J. Mayer-Davis, X. Pi-Sunyer, J. Regensteiner, B. Venditti, and J. Wylie-Rosett, for the Diabetes Prevention Program Research Group. 2006. Effect of weight loss with lifestyle intervention on risk of diabetes. *Diabetes Care* 29(9):2102–2107.

Hampl, S. E., S. G. Hassink, A. C. Skinner, S. C. Armstrong, S. E. Barlow, C. F. Bolling, K. C. Avila Edwards, I. Eneli, R. Hamre, M. M. Joseph, D. Lunsford, E. Mendonca, M. P. Michalsky, N. Mirza, E. R. Ochoa, M. Sharifi, A. E. Staiano, A. E. Weedn, S. K. Flinn, J. Lindros, and K. Okechukwu. 2023. Clinical practice guideline for the evaluation and treatment of children and adolescents with obesity. *Pediatrics* 151(2):e2022060640.

Haqq, A. M., M. Kebbe, Q. Tan, M. Manco, and X. R. Salas. 2021. Complexity and stigma of pediatric obesity. *Child Obesity* 17(4):229–240.

Haynes, A., I. Kersbergen, A. Sutin, M. Daly, and E. Robinson. 2018. A systematic review of the relationship between weight status perceptions and weight loss attempts, strategies, behaviours and outcomes. *Obesity Reviews* 19(3):347–363.

Hazzard, V. M., S. L. Hahn, and K. R. Sonneville. 2017. Weight misperception and disordered weight control behaviors among U.S. high school students with overweight and obesity: Associations and trends, 1999–2013. *Eating Behaviors* 26:189–195.

Healthcare Bluebook. 2023. https://www.healthcarebluebook.com/ui/home (accessed October 20, 2023).

Healthy People 2030. n.d. *Browse Objectives.* https://health.gov/healthypeople/objectives-and-data/browse-objectives (accessed October 20, 2023).

HHS (U.S. Department of Health and Human Services). 2001. *The Surgeon General's Call to Action to Prevent and Decrease Overweight and Obesity.* Rockville, MD: U.S. Department of Health and Human Services, Public Health Service, Office of the Surgeon General. https://www.ncbi.nlm.nih.gov/books/NBK44206/pdf/Bookshelf_NBK44206.pdf (accessed October 20, 2023).

Huizinga, M. M., S. N. Bleich, M. C. Beach, J. M. Clark, and L. A. Cooper. 2010. Disparity in physician perception of patients' adherence to medications by obesity status. *Obesity* 18(10):1932–1937.

Hunger, J. M., and B. Major. 2015. Weight stigma mediates the association between BMI and self-reported health. *Health Psychology* 34(2):172.

IOM (Institute of Medicine). 2012. *Accelerating progress in obesity prevention: Solving the weight of the nation.* Washington, DC: The National Academies Press.

James, W. P. 2008. WHO recognition of the global obesity epidemic. *International Journal of Obesity* 32(Suppl7):S120-6.

Jensen, M. D., D. H. Ryan, C. M. Apovian, J. D. Ard, A. G. Comuzzie, K. A. Donato, F. B. Hu, V. S. Hubbard, J. M. Jakicic, R. F. Kushner, C. M. Loria, B. E. Millen, C. A. Nonas, F. X. Pi-Sunyer, J. Stevens, V. J. Stevens, T. A. Wadden, B. M. Wolfe, and S. Z. Yanovski. 2013. AHA/ACC/TOS guideline for the management of overweight and obesity in adults. *Circulation* 63(25):2985–3023.

Kirk, S. F. L., X. Ramos Salas, A. S. Alberga, and S. Russell-Mayhew. 2020. *Canadian Adult Obesity Clinical Practice Guidelines: Reducing Weight Bias in Obesity Management, Practice and Policy.* https://obesitycanada.ca/guidelines/weightbias (accessed August 9, 2023).

Kling, H. E., X. Yang, S. E. Messiah, K. L. Arheart, D. Brannan, and A. J. Caban-Martinez. 2016. Opportunities for increased physical activity in the workplace: The Walking Meeting (WaM) pilot study, Miami, 2015. *Preventing Chronic Disease* 13(E83).

Kling, H., K. Santiago, L. Benitez, N. Schaefer Solle, and A. J. Caban-Martinez. 2020. Characterizing objective and self-reported levels of physical activity among Florida firefighters across weight status category: A cross-sectional pilot study. *Workplace Health and Safety* 68(11):513–518.

Kuk, J. L., C. I. Ardern, T. S. Church, A. M. Sharma, R. Padwal, X. Sui, and S. N. Blair. 2011. Edmonton Obesity Staging System: Association with weight history and mortality risk. *Applied Physiology, Nutrition, and Metabolism* 36(4):570–576.

Kumanyika, S. 2017. Getting to equity in obesity prevention: A new framework. *NAM Perspectives*. Discussion Paper, National Academy of Medicine, Washington, DC. https://doi.org/10.31478/201701c.

Kumanyika, S. K. 2019. A framework for increasing equity impact in obesity prevention. *American Journal of Public Health* 109:1350–1357.

Kyle, T. K., and R. M. Puhl. 2014. Putting people first in obesity. *Obesity* 22(5):1211.

Kyle, T. K., E. J. Dhurandhar, and D. B. Allison. 2016. Regarding obesity as a disease: Evolving policies and their implications. *Endocrinology and Metabolism Clinics of North America* 45(3):511–520.

MacInnis, C. C., A. S. Alberga, S. Nutter, J. H. Ellard, and S. Russell-Mayhew. 2020. Regarding obesity as a disease is associated with lower weight bias among physicians: A cross-sectional survey study. *Stigma and Health* 5(1):114–122.

Martin, A. B., M. Hartman, J. Benson, A. Catlin, and National Health Expenditure Accounts Team. 2023. National health care spending in 2021: Decline in federal spending outweighs greater use of health care: Study examines national health care expenditures in 2021. *Health Affairs* 42(1):6–17.

Martin, C. B., K. A. Herrick, N. Sarafrazi, and C. L. Ogden. 2018. Attempts to lose weight among adults in the United States, 2013–2016. NCHS Data Brief, no 313. Hyattsville, MD: National Center for Health Statistics.

Martin, C. B., B. Stierman, J. A. Yanovski, C. M. Hales, N. Sarafrazi, and C. L. Ogden. 2022. Body fat differences among U.S. youth aged 8–19 by race and Hispanic origin, 2011–2018. *Pediatric Obesity* 17(7):e12898.

Mechanick, J. I., D. L. Hurley, and W. T. Garvey. 2017. Adiposity-based chronic disease as a new diagnostic term: The American Association of Clinical Endocrinologists and American College of Endocrinology Position Statement. *Endocrine Practice* 23(3):372–378.

Miller, D. P., Jr., J. G. Spangler, M. Z. Vitolins, S. W. Davis, E. H. Ip, G. S. Marion, and S. J. Crandall. 2013. Are medical students aware of their anti-obesity bias? *Academic Medicine* 88(7):978–982.

Minnesota Department of Health. 2021. *SWOT Analysis*. https://www.health.state.mn.us/communities/practice/resources/phqitoolbox/swot.html#:~:text=More%20information-,What%20is%20a%20SWOT%20analysis%3F,weaknesses%2C%20opportunities%2C%20and%20threats (accessed October 20, 2023).

Mylod, D., and T. H. Lee. 2023. Giving hope as a high reliability function of health care. *Journal of Patient Experience* 10:1–3.

NCQA (National Committee for Quality Assurance). 2023. *Adult BMI Assessment*. https://www.ncqa.org/hedis/measures/adult-bmi-assessment (accessed October 20, 2023).

OAC (Obesity Action Coalition). 2023. *Weight Bias Program*. https://www.obesityaction.org/weightbias/#:~:text=The%20OAC%27s%20Weight%20Bias%20Program,tools%20to%20make%20a%20difference (accessed October 20, 2023).

Obesity Medicine Association. 2017. *Definition of Obesity*. https://obesitymedicine.org/definition-of-obesity (accessed October 20, 2023).

OCEANS (Outreach, Community, Engagement, Advocacy, Non-Discriminatory Support). 2023. *@oceanslifestyles*. https://www.instagram.com/oceanslifestyles/?hl=en (accessed October 20, 2023).

Ogden, C. L., C. D. Fryar, C. B. Martin, D. S. Freedman, M. D. Carroll, Q. Gu, and C. M. Hales. 2020. Trends in obesity prevalence by race and Hispanic origin—1999–2000 to 2017–2018. *Journal of the American Medical Association* 324(12):1208–1210.

O'Keeffe, M., S. W. Flint, K. Watts, and F. Rubino. 2020. Knowledge gaps and weight stigma shape attitudes toward obesity. *The Lancet Diabetes and Endocrinology* 8(5):363–365.

O'Rahilly, S. 2021. "Treasure your exceptions"—Studying human extreme phenotypes to illuminate metabolic health and disease: The 2019 Banting Medal for Scientific Achievement Lecture. *Diabetes* 70(1):29–38.

Padwal, R. S., N. M. Pajewski, D. B. Allison, and A. M. Sharma. 2011. Using the Edmonton Obesity Staging System to predict mortality in a population-representative cohort of people with overweight and obesity. *Canadian Medical Association Journal* 183(14):E1059–E1066.

Peretti, J. 2013. Fat profits: How the food industry cashed in on obesity. *The Guardian*, August 7. https://www.theguardian.com/lifeandstyle/2013/aug/07/fat-profits-food-industry-obesity (accessed October 20, 2023).

Phelan, S. M., D. J. Burgess, M. W. Yeazel, W. L. Hellerstedt, J. M. Griffin, and M. van Ryn. 2015. Impact of weight bias and stigma on quality of care and outcomes for patients with obesity. *Obesity Reviews* 16(4): 319–326.

Poston, W. S. C, C. K. Haddock, S. A. Jahnke, N. Jitnarin, B. C. Tuley, and S. N. Kales. 2011. The prevalence of overweight, obesity, and substandard fitness in a population-based firefighter cohort. *Journal of Occupational and Environmental Medicine* 53(3):266–273.

Puhl, R. M. 2020. What words should we use to talk about weight? A systematic review of quantitative and qualitative studies examining preferences for weight-related terminology. *Obesity Reviews* 21:e13008.

Puhl, R. M., and Heuer, C.A. 2009. The stigma of obesity: A review and update. *Obesity* 17(5):941–964.

Puhl, R., and Y. Suh. 2015. Health consequences of weight stigma: Implications for obesity prevention and treatment. *Current Obesity Reports* 4(2):182–190.

Puhl, R. M., M. S. Himmelstein, S. C. Armstrong, and E. Kingsford. 2017. Adolescent preferences and reactions to language about body weight. *International Journal of Obesity* 41(7):1062–1065.

Puhl, R. M., M. S. Himmelstein, and D. M. Quinn. 2018. Internalizing weight stigma: Prevalence and sociodemographic considerations in U.S. adults. *Obesity* 26(1):167–175.

Puhl, R. M., L. M. Lessard, G. D. Foster, and M. I. Cardel. 2022. Patient and family perspectives on terms for obesity. *Pediatrics* 150(6):e2022058204.

Richmond, T. K., I. B. Thurston, and K. R. Sonneville. 2021. Weight-focused public health interventions—no benefit, some harm. *Journal of the American Medical Association Pediatrics* 175(3):238–239.

Roser, M. 2020. *Why Is Life Expectancy in the U.S. Lower Than in Other Rich Countries?* https://ourworldindata.org/us-life-expectancy-low (accessed October 20, 2023).

Rubino, F., R. M. Puhl, D. E. Cummings, R. H. Eckel, D. H. Ryan, J. I. Mechanick, J. Nadglowski, X. Ramos Salas, P. R. Schauer, D. Twenefour, C. M. Apovian, L. J. Aronne, R. L. Batterham, H.-R. Berthoud, C. Boza, L. Busetto, D. Dicker, M. De Groot, D. Eisenberg, S. W. Flint, T. T. Huang, L. M. Kaplan, J. P. Kirwan, J. Korner, T. K. Kyle, B. Laferrère, C. W. le Roux, L. McIver, G. Mingrone, P. Nece, T. J. Reid, A. M. Rogers, M. Rosenbaum, R. J. Seeley, A. J. Torres, and J. B. Dixon. 2020. Joint international consensus statement for ending stigma of obesity. *Nature Medicine* 26(4):485–497.

Rubino, F., R. L. Batterham, M. Koch, G. Mingrone, C. W. le Roux, I. S. Farooqi, N. Farpour-Lambert, E. W. Gregg, and D. E. Cummings. 2023. Lancet Diabetes & Endocrinology Commission on the Definition and Diagnosis of Clinical Obesity. *The Lancet Diabetes & Endocrinology* 11(4):226–228.

RWJF (Robert Wood Johnson Foundation). 2023. *Bridge to health graphic*. https://www.rwjf.org/content/dam/rwjf-web/illustrations/RWJFStructuralRacismBridgesSimple1200_675.png# (accessed November 27, 2023).

Sharma, A. M., and R. F. Kushner. 2009. A proposed clinical staging system for obesity. *International Journal of Obesity* 33(3):289–295.

Smith, D. L., P. C. Fehling, A. Frisch, J. M. Haller, M. Winke, and M. W. Dailey. 2012. The prevalence of cardiovascular disease risk factors and obesity in firefighters. *Journal of Obesity* 2012:908267.

Sonneville, K. R., I. B. Thurston, C. E. Milliren, H. C. Gooding, and T. K. Richmond. 2016a. Weight misperception among young adults with overweight/obesity associated with disordered eating behaviors. *International Journal of Eating Disorders* 49(10):937–946.

Sonneville, K. R., I. B. Thurston, C. E. Milliren, R.C. Kamody, H. C. Gooding, and T. K. Richmond. 2016b. Helpful or harmful? Prospective association between weight misperception and weight gain among overweight and obese adolescents and young adults. *International Journal of Obesity* 40(2):328–332.

Stierman, B., J. Afful, M. D. Carroll, T. C. Chen, O. Davy, S. Fink, C. D. Fryar, Q. Gu, C. M. Hales, J. P. Hughes, Y. Ostchega, R. J. Storandt, and L. A. Akinbami. 2021. National Health and Nutrition Examination Survey 2017–March 2020 prepandemic data files— Development of files and prevalence estimates for selected health outcomes. National Health Statistics Reports no 158. Hyattsville, MD: National Center for Health Statistics.

Streeter, J., M. Roche, and A. Friedlander. 2021. *From Bad to Worse: The Impact of Work-from-Home on Sedentary Behaviors and Exercising.* https://longevity.stanford.edu/wp-content/uploads/2021/05/Sedentary-Brief.pdf (accessed October 20, 2023).

Strings, S. 2019. *Fearing the Black body: The racial origins of fat phobia.* New York: New York University Press.

TFAH (Trust for America's Health). 2022. *The State of Obesity: Better Policies for a Healthier America.* https://www.tfah.org/wp-content/uploads/2022/09/2022ObesityReport_FINAL3923.pdf (accessed October 20. 2023).

TFAH. 2023.*The Impact of Chronic Underfunding on America's Public Health System.* https://www.tfah.org/wp-content/uploads/2023/06/TFAH-2023-PublicHealthFundingFINALc.pdf (accessed October 20, 2023).

Thurston, I. B., K. R. Sonneville, C. E. Milliren, R. C. Kamody, H. C. Gooding, and T. K. Richmond. 2017. Cross-sectional and prospective examination of weight misperception and depressive symptoms among youth with overweight and obesity. *Prevention Science* 18:152–163.

Tomiyama, A. J., D. Carr, E. M. Granberg, B. Major, E. Robinson, A. R. Sutin, and A. Brewis. 2018. How and why weight stigma drives the obesity "epidemic" and harms health. *BMC Medicine* 16(1):123.

Tondt, J., M. Freshwater, S. Christensen, M. Iliakova, E. Weaver, S. Benson-Davies, C. Younglove, S. Afreen, S. Karjoo, N. Khan, D. Thiara, and C. Whittle. 2023. *Obesity Algorithm Slides, Presented by the Obesity Medicine Association.* https://obesitymedicine.org/obesity-algorithm-powerpoint (accessed October 20, 2023).

Tylka, T. L., R. A. Annunziato, D. Burgard, S. Daníelsdóttir, E. Shuman, C. Davis, and R. M. Calogero. 2014. The weight-inclusive versus weight-normative approach to health: Evaluating the evidence for prioritizing well-being over weight loss. *Journal of Obesity.* https://doi.org/10.1155/2014/983495.

UConn Rudd Center for Food Policy and Health. 2017. *Weight Bias: A Policy Brief.* https://uconnruddcenter.org/wp-content/uploads/sites/2909/2020/07/Weight-Bias-Policy-Brief-2017.pdf (accessed October 20, 2023).

Unger, E. S., I. Kawachi, C. E. Milliren, K. R. Sonneville, I. B. Thurston, H. C. Gooding, and T. K. Richmond. 2017. Protective misperception? Prospective study of weight self-perception and blood pressure in adolescents with overweight and obesity. *Journal of Adolescent Health* 60(6):680–687.

Venkat Narayan, K. M., D. Kondal, N. Daya, U. P. Gujral, D. Mohan, S. A. Patel, R. Shivashankar, R. M. Anjana, L. R. Staimez, M. K. Ali, H. H. Chang, M. Kadir, D. Prabhakaran, E. Selvin, V. Mohan, and N. Tandon. 2021. Incidence and pathophysiology of diabetes in South Asian adults living in India and Pakistan compared with US Blacks and Whites. *BMJ Open Diabetes Research and Care* 9:e001927.

Venkat Narayan, K. M., D. Kondal, L. R. Staimez, R. Mohan Anjana, U. Gujral, M. Deepa, S. A. Patel, M. K. Ali, D. Prabhakaran, H. H. Chang, N. Tandon, and V. Mohan. 2022. Natural history of type 2 diabetes in South Asians: Arrow of time. *Diabetes* 71(Suppl_1):1193-P.

Ward, Z. J., S. N. Bleich, M. W. Long, and S. L. Gortmaker. 2021. Association of body mass index with health care expenditures in the United States by age and sex. *PloS One* 16(3):e0247307.

Weight Inclusive Nutrition and Dietetics. 2023. *HAES: From a Social Justice "Movement" to a Framework of Care with Veronica Garnett MS RDN, Foundations of WIND Workshop.* https://www.weightinclusivenutrition.com/foundations-of-weight-inclusive-care (accessed September 15, 2023).

White House. 2022. *Biden–Harris Administration National Strategy on Hunger, Nutrition, and Health.* https://www.whitehouse.gov/wp-content/uploads/2022/09/White-House-National-Strategy-on-Hunger-Nutrition-and-Health-FINAL.pdf (accessed October 20, 2023).

WHO (World Health Organization). 1995. *Physical Status: The Use and Interpretation of Anthropometry—Report of a WHO Expert Committee.* https://apps.who.int/iris/bitstream/handle/10665/37003/WHO_TRS_854.pdf?sequence=1&isAllowed=y (accessed October 20, 2023).

Wilding, J. P. H., and S. Jacob. 2021. Cardiovascular outcome trials in obesity: A review. *Obesity Reviews* 22(1):e13112.

Wilkinson, M. L., A. L. Brown, W. S. C. Poston, C. K. Haddock, S. A. Jahnke, and R. S. Day. 2014. Peer reviewed: Physician weight recommendations for overweight and obese firefighters, United States, 2011–2012. *Preventing Chronic Disease* 11.

Zeng, Q., N. Li, X. F. Pan, L. Chen, and A. Pan. 2021. Clinical management and treatment of obesity in China. *Lancet Diabetes and Endocrinology* 9(6):393–405.

Appendix A

Workshop Agendas

BMI and Beyond: Considering Context in Measuring Obesity and Its Applications

April 4, 2023

AGENDA

10:00 AM   Welcome
Nicolaas (Nico) P. Pronk, HealthPartners Institute, Chair of the Roundtable on Obesity Solutions

SESSION 1—"OBESITY": DEFINITIONS AND PERSPECTIVES
Moderator: *S. Bryn Austin, Harvard T.H. Chan School of Public Health*

10:05   **Presenters**
- *Edward (Ted) Fischer, Vanderbilt University*
- *Katherine Flegal, Stanford University*
- *Donna Ryan, Pennington Biomedical Research Center*

SESSION 2—TENSIONS AND PERSPECTIVES AROUND BMI
Moderator: *Michael G. Knight, The GWU Medical Faculty Associates*

10:40   Panelists
• *Jamy D. Ard, Wake Forest School of Medicine*
• *Cynthia Ogden, Centers for Disease Control and Prevention*
• *Stacy E. Wright, University of Florida*

12:00   Lunch Break

SESSION 3—APPLICATIONS AND USES OF BMI, BODY COMPOSITION, AND BODY FAT DISTRIBUTION
Moderator: *W. Scott Butsch, Cleveland Clinic*

12:45 PM   Presenters
• *Michael D. Jensen, Mayo Clinic*
• *David E. Arterburn, Kaiser Permanente*
• *Alberto Caban-Martinez, University of Miami*
• *Faith Anne Heeren, University of Florida*

2:00   Break

SESSION 4—BEST WAYS GOING FORWARD
Moderator: *Nicolaas (Nico) P. Pronk, HealthPartners Institute, Chair of the Roundtable on Obesity Solutions*

2:15   Presenters
• *S. Bryn Austin, Harvard T.H. Chan School of Public Health*
• *Craig M. Hales, U.S. Food and Drug Administration*
• *Michael G. Knight, The GWU Medical Faculty Associates*

3:00   **Closing Remarks**
Ihuoma Eneli, Nationwide Children's Hospital, Vice Chair of the Roundtable on Obesity Solutions

3:15   **ADJOURN**

Going Beyond BMI: Communicating About Body Weight

June 26, 2023

AGENDA

10:00 AM   Welcome
Ihuoma Eneli, Nationwide Children's Hospital, Vice Chair of the Roundtable on Obesity Solutions

SESSION 1—COMMUNICATING HOW OBESITY IS DEFINED AND DIAGNOSED
Moderator: *W. Scott Butsch, Cleveland Clinic*

10:05   Presenters
- *Francesco Rubino, King's College London*
- *W. Timothy Garvey, University of Alabama at Birmingham*
- *Geoff Ball, University of Alberta*

SESSION 2—INNOVATIONS IN COMMUNICATING ABOUT BODY WEIGHT IN THE CLINIC AND BEYOND
Moderator: *Craig M. Hales, U.S. Food and Drug Administration*

11:20   Panelists
- *Kofi Essel, GWU School of Medicine*
- *Robyn Pashby, DC Health Psychology*

12:00 PM   Lunch Break

SESSION 3—ETHICS AND TRUST IN COMMUNICATING ABOUT THE INTERSECTION OF BODY WEIGHT AND HEALTH
Moderator: *S. Bryn Austin, Harvard T.H. Chan School of Public Health*

12:35   Presenters
- *Tracy Richmond, Boston Children's Hospital*
- *Martin Wilkinson, University of Auckland*
- *Thomas Lee, Press Ganey*

SESSION 4—STRATEGIES FOR IMPROVING COMMUNICATION ABOUT BODY WEIGHT
Moderator: *Ihuoma Eneli, Nationwide Children's Hospital, Vice Chair of the Roundtable on Obesity Solutions*

1:45   Presenters
- *J. Nadine Gracia, Trust for America's Health*
- *Jennie Day-Burget, Robert Wood Johnson Foundation*

SESSION 5—STRATEGIES FOR PROMOTING CHANGE IN CULTURE AND PERCEPTION AROUND BODY WEIGHT
Moderator: *Nicolaas (Nico) P. Pronk, HealthPartners Institute, Chair of the Roundtable on Obesity Solutions*

2:30   Presenters
- *Natalia Slopen, Harvard T.H. Chan School of Public Health*
- *Brian Castrucci, de Beaumont Foundation*

3:05   **Closing Remarks**
Nicolaas (Nico) P. Pronk, HealthPartners Institute, Chair of the Roundtable on Obesity Solutions

3:15   **ADJOURN**

Appendix B

Biographical Sketches of Workshop Speakers and Planning Committee Members

Jamy D. Ard, M.D., is professor in the Department of Epidemiology and Prevention and the Department of Medicine at Wake Forest University School of Medicine. He is also codirector of the Atrium Health Wake Forest Baptist Weight Management Center, directing medical weight-management programs. After his residency, he was selected as a chief resident in internal medicine at Duke. He also received formal training in clinical research as a fellow at the Center for Health Services Research in Primary Care at the Durham VA Medical Center; he participated in a focused research experience on lifestyle interventions for hypertension and obesity at the Duke Hypertension Center. Dr. Ard's research interests include clinical management of obesity and strategies to improve cardiometabolic risk using lifestyle modification. In particular, his work has focused on developing and testing medical strategies to treat obesity in special populations, including African Americans, those with type 2 diabetes, and older adults. Dr. Ard has participated in several major National Institutes of Health (NIH)–funded multicenter trials, including Dietary Approaches to Stop Hypertension (DASH), DASH-sodium, PREMIER, and Weight Loss Maintenance Trial. He has been conducting research on lifestyle modification since 1995 and received research funding from a variety of federal and foundation sources, including NIH and the Robert Wood Johnson Foundatiion (RWJF). His work has been published in numerous scientific journals, and he has been a featured presenter at several national and international conferences and workshops dealing with obesity. Dr. Ard has more than 20 years of experience in clinical nutrition and obesity. Prior to joining the faculty at Wake Forest in 2012, Dr. Ard spent 9 years at the University of Alabama at Birmingham in the

Department of Nutrition Sciences. He has served on several expert panels and guideline development committees, including the National Academies (previously the Institute of Medicine) Committee on Consequences of Sodium Reduction in Populations, American Heart Association/American College of Cardiology/The Obesity Society Guideline Panel on the Identification, Evaluation, and Treatment of Overweight and Obesity in Adults, and American Psychological Association Obesity Guideline Development Panel. He is also on the editorial board for the *American Journal of Clinical Nutrition* and the *International Journal of Obesity*. Dr. Ard is a National Academy of Medicine member. He received an M.D. and completed internal medicine residency training at Duke University Medical Center.

David Arterburn, M.D., M.P.H., FACP, FTOS, FASMBS, is a general internist and a senior investigator at the Kaiser Permanente Washington Health Research Institute and an affiliate professor with the University of Washington's Department of Medicine. The main focus of his research is on identifying safe, effective, and affordable interventions to reduce the medical and psychosocial burden of obesity. Dr. Arterburn was the founding chair of the Health Services Research Section of The Obesity Society, chair of the Adult Obesity Measurement Advisory Panel for the National Committee for Quality Assurance that developed Healthcare Effectiveness Data and Information Set performance measures for obesity, and cochair of the 2013 NIH Symposium on Long-Term Outcomes of Bariatric Surgery. Dr. Arterburn received his M.P.H. in health services from the University of Washington School of Public Health and Community Medicine and his M.D. from the University of Kentucky College of Medicine.

S. Bryn Austin, Sc.D., M.S., is professor in social and behavioral sciences at Harvard T.H. Chan School of Public Health, professor of pediatrics at Harvard Medical School, and research scientist with the Division of Adolescent and Young Adult Medicine at Boston Children's Hospital. She is founding director of STRIPED, based at Harvard Chan and Boston Children's. She was director of fellowship research training for the U.S. Maternal and Children Health Bureau–funded Leadership Education in Adolescent Health training grant at Boston Children's from 1999 to 2020. She is a social epidemiologist and behavioral scientist with a research focus on environmental influences on disordered weight and shape control behaviors and weight stigma and on public health prevention approaches with an emphasis on policy translation research and advocacy. Her research also includes a focus on health inequities, especially those affecting socially and structurally marginalized adolescents based on sexual orientation, gender identity, and race/ethnicity. Dr. Austin has received a number of awards for her research, teaching, and mentorship, including from the Society for Adolescent Health and Medicine and AcademyHealth. She has also received numerous research grants as principal investigator and coinvestigator funded by NIH, Department of Defense, the Centers for Disease Control and Prevention (CDC), and foundations. She is a past president of the Academy for Eating Disorders and Eating Disorders Coalition. She received her B.A. in women's studies and African American studies from Cornell University and her M.A. and Ph.D. in health and social behavior from the Harvard School of Public Health.

Geoff Ball, Ph.D., R.D., is professor and associate chair (research) in the Department of Pediatrics and the Alberta Health Services Chair in Obesity Research in the Faculty of Medicine and Dentistry at the University of Alberta in Edmonton, Canada. He served as the founding director of the Pediatric Centre for Weight and Health (2004–2022), a multidisciplinary obesity management clinic at the Stollery Children's Hospital. His clinical and applied health research applies diverse methods (clinical trials, qualitative research, epidemiology, and knowledge syntheses) to generate, evaluate, and apply new knowledge to optimize obesity management and prevention in children and families. In addition to his successful record in publishing and mentoring learners, Dr. Ball has received support from a range of funding agencies, including the Canadian Institutes of Health Research (continuously since 2003). Dr. Ball has led multiple successful team grants and, in partnership with Obesity Canada, chairs a national committee of parents, clinicians, and researchers to update the Canadian clinical practice guideline for managing pediatric obesity. He received a B.Sc. in dietetics from the University of British Columbia, completed a dietetic internship with Capital Health (Alberta), obtained a Ph.D. in nutrition metabolism from the University of Alberta, and completed postdoctoral training at the University of Southern California.

W. Scott Butsch, M.D., M.Sc., FTOS, has been the director of obesity medicine in the Bariatric and Metabolic Institute at the Cleveland Clinic since 2018. He was on staff at Massachusetts General Hospital and an instructor in medicine at Harvard Medical School from 2008 to 2018; he was one of the first two U.S. physicians to complete a subspecialty fellowship in obesity medicine in 2008 at the hospital and school. Dr. Butsch is a leader in obesity education and has been instrumental in shaping the state of education and training in the United States and abroad. With his idea to create core obesity competencies in U.S. medical schools, Dr. Butsch has helped formalize and expand obesity education in undergraduate and graduate medical education. He has created/cocreated numerous national and international education programs for practitioners. He has authored numerous chapters and manuscripts and lectures nationally and internationally on obesity management. Dr. Butsch has served in the Obesity Medicine Education

Collaborative and Integrated Clinical and Social Systems for the Prevention and Management of Obesity Innovative Collaborative (a satellite activity of the National Academies' Roundtable on Obesity Solutions) specifically to develop core competencies in obesity medicine. Dr. Butsch received his M.D. from the University of Buffalo in 2001. He completed fellowships in clinical nutrition (2007) and medical education (2008) at the University of Alabama at Birmingham and Harvard, respectively. He is a diplomate of the American Board of Obesity Medicine and fellow of The Obesity Society.

Alberto Juan Caban-Martinez, D.O., Ph.D., M.P.H., CPH, is a board-certified physician-scientist, associate professor (tenured) of public health sciences, deputy director of the M.D.-M.P.H. program, and associate provost for regulatory affairs, assessment, and research integrity at the University of Miami. He has more than 10 years of domestic and international research expertise in environmental and occupational epidemiology. He serves as the deputy director of the Firefighter Cancer Initiative at the Sylvester Comprehensive Cancer Center and codirector and principal investigator of the Federal Emergency Management Agency–funded Fire Fighter Cancer Cohort Study, a national epidemiologic study that includes underrepresented firefighter subgroups, such as arson investigators, trainers/instructors, wildland–urban interface firefighters, and volunteers. He is a former fellow of the National Academy of Sciences' Gulf Research Program and served on the IOM Committee on Gulf War and Health for 2 years to provide scientific expertise on occupational exposures and work-related health conditions. His research with first responders and construction workers led him to serve on the National Institute of Occupational Safety and Health National Occupational Research Agenda committee, setting the national research agenda on worker health and safety. He has scientific articles in the *New England Journal of Medicine, JAMA, JAMA Network Open, JAMA Dermatology,* CDC's *Morbidity and Mortality Weekly Report, American Journal of Public Health, Occupational and Environmental Medicine, Preventive Medicine,* and *Neuropharmacology.* He has more than 178 peer-reviewed publications and more than 256 scientific presentations on a wide range of occupational health and safety topics. Dr. Caban-Martinez received his D.O. from Nova Southeastern University College of Osteopathic Medicine and his Ph.D. from the University of Miami, Miller School of Medicine Department of Epidemiology.

Brian C. Castrucci, Dr.P.H., M.A., is president and chief executive officer (CEO) of the de Beaumont Foundation. He has built the foundation into a leading voice in health philanthropy and public health practice. An award-winning epidemiologist with 10 years of experience in the health departments of Philadelphia, Texas, and Georgia, Dr. Castrucci brings a unique perspective to the philanthropic sector that allows him to shape and implement visionary and practical initiatives and partnerships and bring together research and practice to improve public health. Dr. Castrucci holds a Dr.P.H. in public health leadership from the Gillings School of Global Public Health at the University of North Carolina at Chapel Hill and an M.A. in sociomedical sciences from Columbia University.

Jennie Day-Burget is senior communications officer at RWJF, where she splits her time between RWJF's Healthy Communities, childhood obesity and structural racism, and health message research initiatives. She was vice president and managing director at Prichard, a boutique communications agency, where she led its work with RWJF and many of its grantees. She also led communications efforts for nonprofit and foundation clients, including the Northwest Health Foundation, Meyer Memorial Trust, National Association of Clean Water Agencies, and Communications Network. She led several media relations and public outreach initiatives in her role as a public information officer for the city of Portland, Oregon. Ms. Day-Burget earned a B.A. in English and a B.S. in journalism from the University of Kansas.

Ihuoma Eneli, M.D., M.S., FAAP, (Cochair) is a board-certified general pediatrician. She is section head for nutrition and professor of pediatrics at University of Denver and Children's Hospital Colorado. She was professor of pediatrics at the Ohio State University and director of Nationwide Children's Hospital (NCH) Center for Healthy Weight and Nutrition, Columbus, Ohio. Dr. Eneli is a leader in pediatric obesity. She developed an internationally recognized tertiary care pediatric obesity center with activities that include advocacy, prevention, medical weight management, bariatric surgery, and research. She served as codirector of the NCH Childhood Obesity and Bariatric Surgery Fellowship, the only pediatric fellowship that trains both bariatric surgeons and pediatricians. In 2021, she was awarded the prestigious National Academic Pediatric Association Healthcare Delivery Award in recognition of her work on childhood obesity. She coauthored the 2023 American Academy of Pediatrics (AAP) Clinical Practice Guideline on Childhood Obesity. Her research interest is on interventions for pediatric obesity, for which she has received funding from several sources, including NIH and Patient-Centered Outcomes Research Institute. She has served in leadership and advisory roles for several organizations, including the AAP, National Academies, and Children's Hospital Association. She is an associate director for the AAP Institute for Healthy Childhood Weight and vice chair of the National Academies' Roundtable on Obesity Solutions. Dr. Eneli received her M.D. from University of Nigeria. She completed her pediatric residency and M.S. in epidemiology at Michigan State University.

Kofi D. Essel, M.D., M.P.H., FAAP, is a board-certified community pediatrician at Children's National Hospital in Washington, DC. Dr. Essel serves as assistant professor of pediatrics and director of the George Washington University (GWU) School of Medicine and Health Sciences Culinary Medicine Program, Community/Urban Health Scholarly Concentration, and Clinical Public Health Summit on Obesity. Dr. Essel has recently accepted a role and will be the inaugural food as medicine program director at Elevance Health. He sits on the National Academies' Roundtable on Obesity Solutions' Lived Experience Innovation Collaborative and was nationally recognized by the Alliance for a Healthier Generation for helping to create an innovative curriculum to enhance pediatric resident trainee skills on nutrition-related disease management. He is on the board of directors for the Food Research and Action Center (FRAC) and physician advisor for the Partnership for a Healthier America's "Veggies Early & Often" campaign. Dr. Essel is a member of the executive committee for the AAP Section on Obesity. He also coauthored a national toolkit for pediatric providers to address food insecurity in their clinical settings with AAP and FRAC. Dr. Essel earned a B.S. from Emory University with a focus on human biology/anthropology and his M.D. and M.P.H. in epidemiology from GWU.

Edward (Ted) Fischer, Ph.D., is the Cornelius Vanderbilt Professor of Anthropology, Management, and Health Policy at Vanderbilt University, where he also directs the Cultural Contexts of Health and Well-Being Initiative. In 2009, Dr. Fischer founded Maní+, a successful social enterprise in Guatemala that develops and produces locally sourced foods to fight malnutrition. He advises the World Health Organization on behavioral and cultural insights, and his research focuses on values, well-being, and the political economy of food. He has authored or edited a number of books, including *The Good Life*, and, most recently, *Making Better Coffee: How Maya Farmers and Third Wave Tastemakers Create Value*. He received his Ph.D. from Tulane University.

Katherine Flegal, Ph.D., M.P.H., is a consulting professor at Stanford University. She was a senior scientist at the CDC National Center for Health Statistics. She worked in the biostatistics department of the University of Michigan before joining CDC. Dr. Flegal is one of the most cited scientists in the field of obesity epidemiology. She completed her Ph.D. and M.A. at Cornell University and M.P.H. at the University of Pittsburgh.

W. Timothy Garvey, M.D., is professor of medicine in the Department of Nutrition Sciences at the University of Alabama at Birmingham. He has achieved international recognition for his research in the metabolic, molecular, and genetic pathogenesis of insulin resistance, type 2 diabetes, and obesity. His studies have involved the cellular and molecular biology of cell and animal models, metabolic investigations of human subjects on metabolic research wards, and the genetic basis of diseases in Gullah-speaking African Americans, Pima Indians, and national cohorts of diabetes patients. He has brought basic technology directly to the study of human patients, and the combined approach of human physiology, genetics, and basic cell and molecular biology has provided the laboratory with a flexible capability for hypothesis testing relevant to human disease. Dr. Garvey also has performed community-based research and outreach in the context of two initiatives, Project Sugar (a genetics study among Gullah-speaking African Americans) and MUSC/HBCU Partners in Wellness (a program in community health at six historically Black colleges and universities in South Carolina intended to challenge minority students to join careers in the health professions). He has provided service as a member of national research review committees for the Juvenile Diabetes Research Foundation, American Diabetes Association, VA Merit Review Program, and NIH. He was a standing member of the NIH Metabolism Study Section (1998–2002) and chaired several ad hoc NIH study sections. He is a member of the American Society for Clinical Investigation, Association of American Physicians, Endocrine Society, American Diabetes Association, and North American Association for the Study of Obesity. He obtained his M.D., cum laude, from St. Louis University in 1978 and completed residency in internal medicine at Barnes Hospital, Washington University, in 1981. He was a clinical fellow in endocrinology and metabolism at the University of Colorado Health Sciences Center and University of California, San Diego School of Medicine.

J. Nadine Gracia, M.D., M.S.C.E., is president and CEO and was executive vice president and chief operating officer of Trust for America's Health (TFAH), a nonprofit, nonpartisan public health policy, research, and advocacy organization in Washington, DC, committed to promoting optimal health for every person and community and making prevention and health equity foundational to policymaking at all levels. Dr. Gracia is a national health equity leader with extensive leadership experience in federal government, the nonprofit sector, academia, and professional associations. Before TFAH, Dr. Gracia served in the Obama Administration as the Deputy Assistant Secretary for Minority Health and director of the Department of Health and Human Services (HHS) Office of Minority Health, where she directed departmental policies and programs to end health disparities and advance health equity and provided executive leadership on administration priorities, including the Affordable Care Act and My Brother's Keeper. She was chief medical officer in the HHS Office of the Assistant Secretary for Health, where her portfolio included adolescent health, emergency preparedness, environmental health and climate change, global health, and the White House Council on Women and Girls. Before that, she was a White House Fellow at HHS and worked in the Office of the First Lady on the development of the *Let's Move!* initiative to solve childhood obesity. A first-generation Haitian American, Dr. Gracia is active in many civic, professional, and academic organizations. She is a member of the Aspen Global Leadership Network, National Academy of Medicine Culture of Health Program Advisory Committee, Dean's Council at the University of Maryland School of Public Health, Board of Advisors of the Center for Climate, Health, and Global Environment at the Harvard T.H. Chan School of Public Health, and Women of Impact. Dr. Gracia received her M.D. from the University of Pittsburgh School of Medicine, M.S. in clinical epidemiology from University of Pennsylvania, and B.A. in French from Stanford.

Craig M. Hales, M.D., M.P.H., M.S., is a clinical reviewer with the U.S. Food and Drug Administration Division of Diabetes, Lipid Disorders, and Obesity. Dr. Hales worked with NHANES (2015–2022), where he focused on obesity surveillance and epidemiology. He has coauthored peer-reviewed articles on trends in body composition changes over time and by race and ethnicity using NHANES DEXA scan data. He published a 2022 CDC report recommending the extended method for calculating BMI-for-age percentiles and Z-scores above the 95th percentile, including new versions of the BMI-for-age growth charts for children and adolescents with severe obesity. Dr. Hales is a preventive medicine physician and diplomate of the American Board of Obesity Medicine and practiced at the Johns Hopkins Healthful Eating, Activity, and Weight Program (2020–2022). He also holds M.A. degrees in public health and biostatistics from Johns Hopkins Bloomberg School of Public Health and Georgia State University, respectively. He received his M.D. from Northwestern University Feinberg School of Medicine.

Faith Anne Heeren is a 4th-year doctoral student in the Department of Health Outcomes and Biomedical Informatics at the University of Florida. Mrs. Heeren is also the founder and president of OCEANS, a nonprofit advocacy group for adolescents with obesity. As a teenager, she underwent gastric bypass surgery. Through her preoperative experience, she discovered a passion for patient advocacy and a strong desire to contribute to research. Mrs. Heeren has participated in patient advocacy efforts by serving on the membership committee for the Obesity Action Coalition and sharing her story with several news organizations, including the *New York Times* and *Associated Press*. She has contributed to several research projects at the University of North Carolina at Chapel Hill, Duke University, and the University of Florida during her undergraduate and graduate years. Her research interests include the implementation of evidence-based treatments for obesity and adolescent bariatric surgery patients and programs.

Michael D. Jensen, M.D., holds the Tomas J. Watson, Jr. Professorship in Honor of Dr. Robert L. Frye at the Mayo College of Medicine and is a consultant in the Division of Endocrinology and Metabolism. His clinical interests are primarily focused on obesity and diabetes. Dr. Jensen's research involves the study of human body fat distribution and fatty acid/energy metabolism, focusing specifically on the effects of obesity and body fat distribution on health. NIH has funded his studies for 35 consecutive years. Dr. Jensen was cochair of the NHLBI Expert Panel on the Identification, Evaluation, and Treatment of Overweight and Obesity in Adults (2008–2013) and is the editor in chief of *Obesity*. He has published more than 300 original research articles and more than 80 invited papers and book chapters. Dr. Jensen received his M.D. from the University of Missouri–Kansas City and completed his internal residency medicine and subspecialty training in endocrinology and metabolism at Mayo Clinic, Rochester, Minnesota.

Nathaniel Kendall-Taylor, Ph.D., is CEO of the FrameWorks Institute, a research think tank in Washington, DC. He leads a multidisciplinary team in researching public understanding and framing of social issues and supporting nonprofit organizations to implement findings. A psychological anthropologist, Dr. Kendall-Taylor publishes widely on communications research in the popular and professional press and lectures frequently in the United States and abroad. He is a senior fellow at the Center on the Developing Child at Harvard, visiting professor at the Child Study Center at Yale School of Medicine, and fellow at the British-American Project. Dr. Kendall-Taylor received his M.A. in anthropology and Ph.D. from UCLA.

Michael G. Knight, M.D., M.S.H.P., FACP, Dipl. ABOM, is an internal medicine and obesity medicine physician, associate chief quality and population health officer, head of health care delivery transformation, and medical director of community primary care at the George Washington (GW) Medical Faculty Associates. He is also an assistant professor of medicine at the GWU School of Medicine and Health Sciences. Dr. Knight is board certified in internal medicine and obesity medicine. He practices clinically in the GW General Internal Medicine Practice and Weight Management Clinic, where he works with a multidisciplinary team to provide medical weight management through nutrition, physical activity, and pharmacotherapy. He has received numerous awards for his professional and clinical practice, including the AMA Foundation Leadership Award, Washingtonian Magazine's Top Doctors Award, and Top 40 Under 40 Leaders in Health Award by the National Minority Quality Forum. He completed undergraduate studies at

Oakwood University and attended the Cleveland Clinic Lerner College of Medicine of Case Western Reserve University. Dr. Knight completed residency at New York Presbyterian–Weill Cornell Medical Center and was an RWJF Clinical Scholar at the University of Pennsylvania, where he earned an M.A. in health policy research.

Thomas Lee, M. Sc., M.D., is an internist at Brigham and Women's Hospital in Boston, Massachusetts, and the chief medical officer to Press Ganey, Inc. Before joining Press Ganey in 2013, Dr. Lee was network president for Partners Healthcare System, the integrated delivery system founded by Brigham and Women's and Massachusetts General Hospitals. Dr. Lee has performed research leading to more than 300 articles in peer-reviewed journals and three books. He became a professor at Harvard School of Public Health in 2004. He is a member of the editorial board of *The New England Journal of Medicine*, board of directors of Geisinger Health System and Health Leads, and Panel of Health Advisors of the Congressional Budget Office. He received his B.A. from Harvard College (1975) and M.D. from Cornell University Medical College (1979) and trained in internal medicine and then cardiology at Brigham and Women's Hospital. He received an M.Sc. in epidemiology from Harvard School of Public Health in 1987.

Cynthia Ogden, Ph.D., is an epidemiologist at the National Center for Health Statistics, CDC, overseeing the analysis group within National Health and Nutrition Examination Survey. Her research interests relate to nutrition, particularly growth and obesity. She worked on the 2000 CDC growth charts for children and the recent extended CDC body mass index (BMI) growth charts. Dr. Ogden has published extensively and given numerous presentations on U.S. obesity and dietary intake. She joined CDC as a member of the Epidemic Intelligence Service. Before that, she was in the Nutrition Division at the New York State Department of Health, where she researched obesity among schoolchildren in New York counties. She has also worked on nutrition-related projects for the Food and Agriculture Organization of the United Nations and is an adjunct professor at the Milken Institute School of Public Health, GWU, where she teaches obesity epidemiology. She earned her M.A. and Ph.D. from Cornell University, where her research focused on malnutrition among young children in Kigali, Rwanda.

Robyn Pashby, Ph.D., is a clinical health psychologist who specializes in the cognitive, behavioral, and emotional aspects of health behavior change. Dr. Pashby is experienced in evidence-based interventions for eating and weight concerns, including interpersonal psychotherapy and cognitive behavioral therapy. Her clinical specialization is in the psychological treatment of obesity, binge eating disorder, internalized weight bias, pre- and post-bariatric surgery concerns, and anti-obesity medications. Dr. Pashby is the owner and director of DC Health Psychology, a group health practice in Washington, DC, that offers telehealth therapy nationwide. She also serves on the National Board of Directors of the Obesity Action Coalition. She has presented research and clinical trainings at both national and international conferences, including the Society of Behavioral Medicine, Eating Disorders Research Society, Obesity Action Coalition Your Weight Matters Conference, International Conference on Eating Disorders, Health Disparities and Social Justice Conference, and Annual Australian Universities Community Engagement Alliance National Conference. She served as the assistant director and senior psychologist for the National Center for Weight and Wellness and a consulting psychologist at the GWU Weight Management Program. She was on the board of the Washington, DC, Psychological Association and an advisory board member for the Making Our Vitality Evident program at the Mautner Project in DC designed to support sexual minority women in health behavior changes to reduce obesity. Dr. Pashby earned her Ph.D. in both medical and clinical psychology from the Uniformed Services University of the Health Sciences, F. Edward Hebert Medical School, where she also completed her postdoctoral fellowship in its Eating Behavior Lab. Her postdoctoral training was at the Washington, DC, Veterans Hospital.

Nicolaas (Nico) P. Pronk, Ph.D., M.A., FACSM, FAWHP, (Cochair) is president of the HealthPartners Institute and chief science officer at HealthPartners, Inc. and affiliate professor of health policy and management at the University of Minnesota School of Public Health. HealthPartners Institute is one of the largest medical research and education centers in the Midwest. HealthPartners, Inc., founded in 1957 as a cooperative, is an integrated, nonprofit, member-governed health system providing health care services and health plan financing and administration. Dr. Pronk's work is focused on connecting evidence of effectiveness with the practical application of programs and practices, policies, and systems that measurably improve population health and well-being. His work applies to the workplace, care delivery setting, and community and involves developing new models to improve health and well-being at the research, practice, and policy levels. His research interests include workplace health and safety, obesity, physical activity, and systems approaches to population health and well-being. Dr. Pronk was cochair of the U.S. Secretary of HHS Advisory Committee on National Health Promotion and Disease Prevention Objectives for 2030 ("Healthy People 2030"). He was a member of the Community Preventive Services Task Force and Defense Health Board (formerly "Armed Forces Epidemiological Board") and the founding and past president of the International Association for Worksite Health Promotion and serves on boards and committees at the National Academies and the Health Enhancement Research Organization, among others. Dr. Pronk is a member of the Food and Nutrition Board and chair of the National Academies' Roundtable on Obesity Solutions. Dr. Pronk received his Ph.D. in exercise physiology at Texas A&M University and completed his postdoctoral studies in behavioral medicine at the University of Pittsburgh Medical Center at the Western Psychiatric Institute and Clinic in Pittsburgh, Pennsylvania.

Tracy Richmond, M.D., M.P.H., is director of the Boston Children's Hospital Eating Disorders Program and the STEP program, a multidisciplinary program focused on the wellness of youth with elevated BMIs, many of whom have disordered eating. Dr. Richmond is a clinician researcher trained in pediatrics and adolescent medicine and social epidemiology (through the RWJF Clinical Scholars Program) with 20 years' experience conducting weight and eating disorder research while also providing care to a diverse population of adolescents. In addition to primary and subspecialty reproductive endocrinology care, she cares for patients struggling with issues across the weight spectrum. In her own practice, she treats patients with the full range of weight-related issues, from youth with higher weights to those with restrictive eating disorders. She serves as the research director of the National Eating Disorder Quality Improvement Collaborative, a group of 20+ academic adolescent medicine programs focused on improving care, and cochaired the International Consortium on Health Outcome Measurement's Eating Disorder Outcomes set development. Dr. Richmond earned her M.P.H. from the University of Michigan and her M.D. from the Medical School at the University of Cincinnati and completed her residency in pediatrics at the University of Michigan.

Francesco Rubino, M.D., is a leading, internationally renowned bariatric surgeon and a pioneer in the field of metabolic weight-loss treatment and surgery, based in London. Dr. Rubino became chief of gastrointestinal metabolic surgery and director of the Diabetes Surgery Centre at Weill Cornell Medical College while also serving as an attending surgeon at New York Presbyterian Hospital in New York. His surgery training was furthered during his fellowship in laparoscopic and minimally invasive surgery at the European Institute of Telesurgery in Strasbourg, France, Mount Sinai Medical Center in New York, and Cleveland Clinic in Ohio. Dr. Rubino has transformed bariatrics from weight-loss therapy to a surgical treatment for multiple metabolic conditions. He received his M.D. and completed his residency in general surgery at the Catholic University in Rome, Italy.

Donna Ryan, M.D., is professor emerita at Pennington Biomedical in Baton Rouge, Louisiana, where she oversaw clinical research for 25 years. Dr.

Ryan's research interests involve lifestyle modification and diet for weight loss and extend to studying the use of medications and devices to aid weight management. She was an investigator on NIH studies, such as the POUNDS (Preventing Overweight Using Novel Dietary Strategies) Lost study, the Look AHEAD (Action for Health in Diabetes) trial, the Diabetes Prevention Program, and DASH. Dr. Ryan also served as principal investigator for the U.S. Department of Defense for a series of awards that targeted military nutrition approaches to improve soldier readiness and performance. A particular research interest was improving primary care management of obesity and evaluating commercial approaches to weight management. Dr. Ryan was president of The Obesity Society and designated Master of Obesity Medicine by the American Board of Obesity Medicine. She serves as publications committee chair following her tenure as past president of the World Obesity Federation. She is also cochair of the Semaglutide Effects on Cardiovascular Outcomes in People with Overweight or Obesity Steering Committee and member of the Data Safety Monitoring Boards for setmelanotide and retatrutide. Dr. Ryan has more than 300 publications and is an active consultant and advisor to companies developing drugs, devices, lifestyle programs, and medical approaches to obesity management. She received her M.D. from Louisiana State University School of Medicine, New Orleans, where she completed her internship at its Charity Hospital and fellowship in medical oncology at its Department of Medicine, Hematology/Medical Oncology Section. She was mentored by George Bray, M.D., when she changed careers to engage in clinical research in obesity.

Natalie Slopen, Sc.D., is assistant professor in the Department of Social and Behavioral Sciences at Harvard T.H. Chan School of Public Health and an affiliated faculty member at the Center on the Developing Child at Harvard. With over a decade of experience as a social epidemiologist, Dr. Slopen is a recognized expert on topics related to the social and environmental determinants of children's health and health disparities. Dr. Slopen leads an interdisciplinary research program focused on the early life origins of racial/ethnic and socioeconomic health disparities, with an emphasis on determinants of health that can be targeted by social policies to advance health equity. She has published her work in peer-reviewed journals on topics related to neighborhoods, housing, economic strain, and traumatic experiences, including empirical studies and systematic review articles. In 2019, Dr. Slopen served on the National Academies committee that produced *Vibrant and Healthy Kids: Aligning Science, Practice, and Policy to Advance Health Equity*. She earned her B.Sc. in psychology from the University of Toronto, M.A. of social sciences from the University of Chicago, and Sc.D. in social epidemiology from the Harvard T.H. Chan School of Public Health.

Martin Wilkinson, M.A., D.Phil., is professor of politics and international relations at the University of Auckland, where he teaches and writes on political theory and public health ethics. He was a senior lecturer and then associate professor in the university's School of Population Health (2003–2009), chair of New Zealand's Bioethics Council and deputy chair of the National Ethics Advisory Committee (two ministerial advisory committees) (2002–2016), and member of Ministry of Health Expert Advisory Groups. He is on the Auckland Hospital Clinical Ethics committee. Dr. Wilkinson received his B.A. and Ph.D. from Oxford University.

Stacy E. Wright, M.P.H., CHES, is pursuing her Ph.D. in health outcomes and implementation science at the University of Florida. Her research areas of interest are obesity and weight stigma among Black women. She was born and raised in Jamaica. For more than 28 years, she was significantly impacted by obesity, low self-esteem, teasing, and discrimination. She wanted nothing more than to lose weight, and she tried all the fad diets but inevitably failed. After years of struggling with her weight and concern for her health and the need for more health education in Jamaica, Ms. Wright obtained her M.A. in public health with a specialization in community health and became a certified health education specialist. She is also a lifestyle advocate; that inspired her first book, *The Healthy Makeover,* which chronicles her 100-pound weight-loss story and the impact of obesity on self-esteem, dieting, facts about hypertension and obesity, and strategies she used to lose weight. Her long-term goal is to create interventions to support individuals and minoritized populations to effectively manage, reduce, and treat obesity. Ms. Wright has work experience in the United States, Japan, and Jamaica. Her most recent position was communications officer/research writer in the Health Promotion and Education Unit within the Ministry of Health in Jamaica.